Acknowledgements

We are grateful to the following for providing some of the illustrations for this book: Sir John Dewhurst, Dr. R.J.S. Harris, Dr. J. Robinson, Mr. D.H. Oram, Dr. S. Thorpe, Dr. P. Greenhouse, Dr. C. Watson, Miss M. Hooper, Dr. S. Barton, Dr. R. Jelley, Mr. R. Forman, Dr. I. Fogelman, Dr. C. Brown, Mr. E. Versi, Dr. F. Mitchell, Mr. M. Emens; Duphar, Serono, Sandoz Pharmaceutical Laboratories, The Royal College of Surgeons, and Gower Medical Publishing. We would especially like to thank Dr. Jo Rosenthal for reading the scripts and providing useful criticisms. We are indebted to the photographic departments of Guy's Hospital and the Royal London Hospital.

Contents

1 / Making a gynaecological diagnosis

History

A thorough history is essential to make an accurate gynaecological diagnosis.

Setting The setting for the interview should ensure privacy and comfort for the woman, who should not be asked to undress before being interviewed (Fig. 1).

Content Specific information should be gathered regarding:

- parity
- last menstrual period
- length of the menstrual cycle
- contraceptive use
- date of the last cervical smear.

The presenting complaint should be clearly defined and put in the context of the previous obstetric and gynaecological history. It is important to record information about sexual activity: duration of the present sexual relationship and any recent change in sexual partner. In cases of suspected infection it is mandatory to ask about the symptoms of the partner(s).

Examination

Positions A pelvic examination can be performed with the patient either in the dorsal position or in the left lateral position (Figs 2 & 3). Sim's position, which is similar to the coma position, may also be used. In the dorsal position the external genitalia are easily inspected, with particular reference to the vulva, labia, clitoris and urethra.

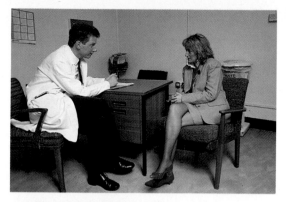

Fig. 1 Gynaecology consultation.

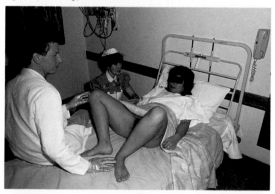

Fig. 2 Examination in the dorsal position.

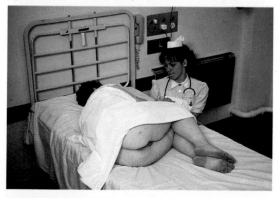

Fig. 3 Patient in the left lateral position.

Bivalve speculum A bivalve speculum is used to inspect the cervix and the vaginal walls (Fig. 4). It is also used when taking cervical smears and endocervical swabs.

Bimanual examination A bimanual examination is performed to assess the pelvic organs. One or two fingers of the right hand are inserted into the vagina and used to elevate and steady the uterus and adnexa so that the left hand on the abdomen can feel the pelvic organs (Fig. 5). The size, position (anteverted, axial or retroverted) and mobility of the uterus are determined together with the presence of tendernes and/or masses in the fornices. *Cervical excitation* is defined as tenderness which arises in one or other adnexum when the broad ligament is stretched by movement of the cervix with the examining fingers.

Sim's speculum The left lateral position facilitates the use of a Sim's speculum (Fig. 6). This instrument was originally designed for displaying vesicovaginal fistulae. It is now more often used in the asessment of uterovaginal prolapse. One end of the speculum is inserted into the vagina and gentle traction applied backwards. The anterior vaginal wall is thus visualized. To view the posterior vaginal wall, a pair of sponge-holding forceps are inserted to retract the anterior vaginal wall while the Sims speculum is slowly withdrawn.

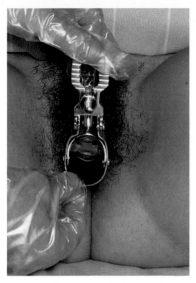

Fig. 4 Examination with a bivalve speculum.

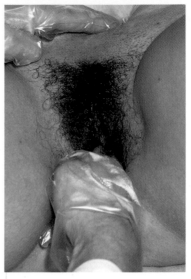

Fig. 5 Bimanual examination.

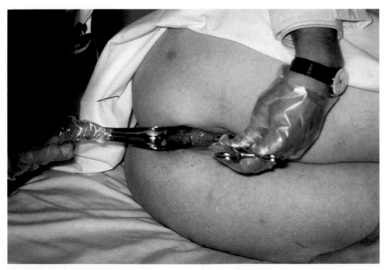

Fig. 6 Examination using Sims speculum.

2 / Investigative techniques

Taking a cervical smear

The cervix should be clearly visualized using a bivalve speculum. The narrow point of the wooden spatula is inserted into the endocervical canal so that the lip rests against the cervix (Fig. 7). It is then rotated through 360 degrees, keeping in firm contact with the cervix, and then removed. The material collected on the spatula is spread evenly on a microscope slide (Fig. 8) which is immediately immersed in fixative (3% acetic acid in 95% alcohol).

Indications All sexually active women should have smears taken at three-yearly intervals.

Taking microbiological swabs

High vaginal swabs are taken from the posterior fornix using a bivalve speculum. The cotton-tipped swab is placed in the appropriate transport medium.

Indications High vaginal swabs are used to detect lower genital tract pathogens, e.g. *Candida albicans* or *Trichomonas vaginalis*, which give rise to symptoms such as discharge and vulval irritation. Endocervical swabs are used to detect pathogens which may spread to the upper genital tract and cause pelvic inflammatory disease, e.g. *Chlamydia trachomatis* and *Neisseria gonorrhoeae*. These bacteria infect columnar epithelium. The microbiological swab should be inserted into the endocervical canal (Fig. 9), agitated and withdrawn. It should then be placed in the appropriate transport medium.

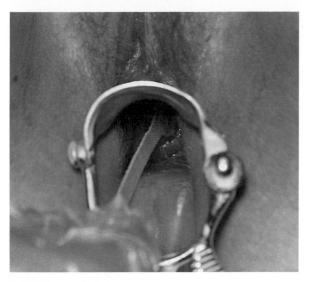

Fig. 7 Taking a cervical smear.

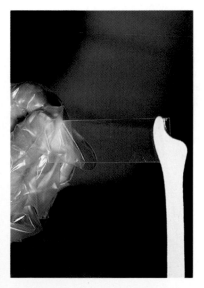

Fig. 8 Spreading the smear on a microscope slide.

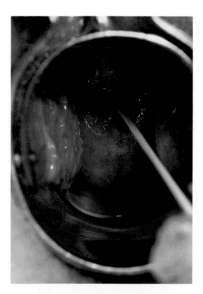

Fig. 9 Taking an endocervical swab.

Colposcopy

Indications   All women who have had cervical smears showing mild dyskaryosis which does not resolve spontaneously, or those women with a single smear showing moderately or severely dyskariotic cells, should undergo colposcopy.

Description   The colposcope (Fig. 10) is a binocular microscope. An illuminated, three-dimensional view of the cervix is obtained, magnified between 6 and 40 times (Fig. 11). This technique identifies both the severity of the abnormality giving rise to an abnormal smear and also its position on the cervix. Hence, it allows the clinician to assess the suitability for local ablative therapy.

Technique   The patient is examined in the lithotomy position, and a bivalve speculum is used to expose the cervix. A further cervical smear is usually taken prior to the colposcopic examination. Cotton wool swabs are then used to clean mucus off the cervix before applying 5% acetic acid to stain the abnormal areas white (acetowhite). If the upper limit of the transformation zone lies within the endocervical canal, forceps may be useful in exposing the whole area (Fig. 12). If the upper limit of the transformation zone cannot be visualized then the examination must be considered incomplete. This occurs in less than 10% of women aged 25 years or less, but in more than 30% of women over the age of 40 years.

Punch biopsy forceps are used to obtain specimens from abnormal areas if the whole of the transformation zone has been visualized. These are sent for histological analysis. An alternative is to undertake a shallow cone biopsy using laser or a diathermy loop.

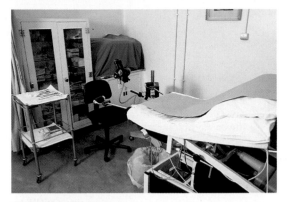

Fig. 10 Colposcopy clinic.

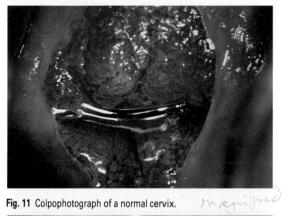

Fig. 11 Colpophotograph of a normal cervix.   magnified 6–40 times

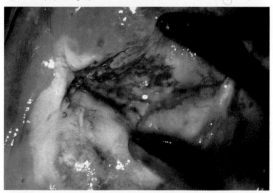

Fig. 12 Exposing the squamocolumnar junction.

Ultrasound

Description Ultrasonography records high-frequency sound waves as they are reflected from anatomic structures. Ultrasound waves are mechanical waves beyond the scope of hearing. When they are directed toward media of differing densities, the sound waves spread out with differing velocities. Echoes arise at the interfaces between these media, and the greater the density differences the greater the intensity of the echoes. This echo signal is measured and converted into a clinical picture of the area under examination. Thus, for good visualization there must be an air-free coupling of the transducer to the abdomen. Ultrasound is a simple and painless procedure that has no known ill-effects. The ultrasonographer and patient can look at the ultrasound image together (Fig. 13).

Various probes are now available (Fig. 14). If an abdominal probe is used, the scan is performed with a full bladder which provides a sonographic 'window'. A vaginal probe eliminates the need to have a full bladder, which is especially useful in early pregnancy.

Indications Ultrasonography is useful in almost any pelvic abnormality as all structures can usually be demonstrated, except in very obese women. Blood flow to various organs can be demonstrated using Colour Doppler techniques (Fig. 15).

The first sign of an intrauterine pregnancy can be detected in the fifth week as a small, sharply outlined cavity which is the gestational sac. Between the 7th and 8th week, embryonic structures can be visualized as distinct echoes and the fetal heart can be seen beating.

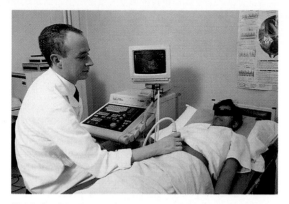

Fig. 13 An abdominal ultrasound being performed.

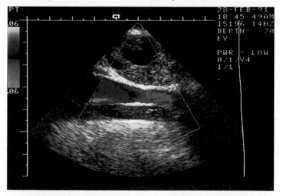

Fig. 14 Vaginal and abdominal ultrasound probes.

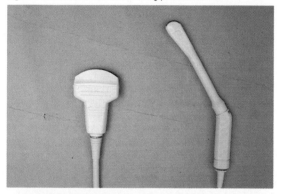

Fig. 15 Colour Doppler ultrasound illustrating normal ovarian blood flow.

Hysterosalpingography

Description   Hysterosalpingography (HSG) is an X-ray method of assessing fallopian tube patency and demonstrating structural abnormalities of the uterine cavity.

Indications   HSG will show whether the fallopian tubes are patent. If not, the area in which the tubes are blocked can be identified. It will not give information concerning the condition of the pelvis, i.e. the presence of peritubular adhesions and/or pelvic distortion which may impair fertility even though the tubes are patent.

Technique   HSG is usually performed without anaesthetic in the X-ray department. A bivalve speculum is used to expose the cervix which is cannulated to enable radiopaque dye to be injected into the uterine cavity. The procedure is viewed using an image intensifier and recorded on film (Fig. 16).

Hysteroscopy

Description and technique   Hysteroscopy is a method which enables visual examination of the uterine cavity. A hysteroscope is a telescope surrounded by a sheath (Fig. 17). It is inserted into the uterine cavity through the cervix with the patient in the lithotomy position and under either local or general anaesthesia.

Indications   Endometrial polyps, fibroids and adhesions within the uterine cavity can be visualized hysteroscopically, together with different types of endometrium e.g. normal, hyperplastic, atrophic and malignant. It is also possible to use the hysteroscope to take endometrial biopsies, divide adhesions and remove the endometrial lining by laser or electrocautery.

Complications   Complications of the procedure include perforation of the uterus, infection and fluid overload (e.g. if fluid distension medium is used for endometrial resection).

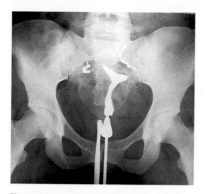

Fig. 16 Hysterosalpingogram outlining the uterine and tubal anatomy.

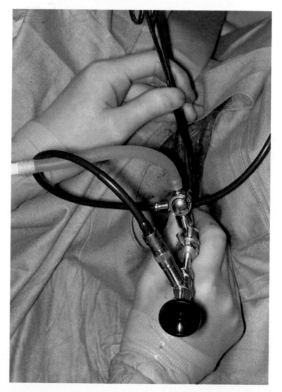

Fig. 17 Diagnostic hysteroscopy (liquid distension medium).

Laparoscopy

Description   The laparoscope (Fig. 18) is essentially a telescope which is inserted into the abdominal cavity after it has been inflated with carbon-dioxide. The direct view obtained allows the diagnosis of gynaecological disorders and limited surgery (Fig. 19) without laparotomy.

Technique   The procedure is almost invariably performed under general anaesthesia with the patient paralysed and ventilated. The patient is placed in the modified Lloyd–Davies position with the head down. The bladder is catheterized. A small incision is made at the umbilicus and a Verre's needle is inserted into the peritoneal cavity. Approximately 3 litres of carbon dioxide are insufflated into the peritoneal cavity. The needle is withdrawn and the laparoscopic trocar and cannula inserted. The trocar is withdrawn and replaced with the laparoscope which allows direct visualization of the pelvic organs (Fig. 20). If needed, further cannulae are inserted under direct laparoscopic vision, suprapubically or in either iliac fossa, to permit manipulation of pelvic organs and instrumentation for various surgical techniques.

Indications   These include pelvic pain, exclusion of ectopic pregnancy, infertility, sterilization, trauma, lost IUCD and assisted conception techniques.

Complications   Complications of the procedure include:
- pain, especially shoulder tip pain from CO_2 diaphragmatic irritation
- bleeding
- puncture of bladder, bowel
- misplacement of gas.

There is a mortality rate of approximately 1 in 15 000.

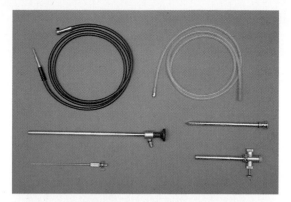

Fig. 18 Instruments used for laparoscopy.

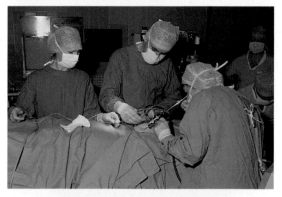

Fig. 19 Laparoscopic aspiration of an ovarian cyst.

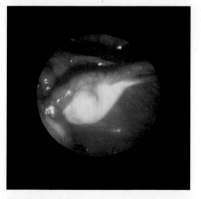

Fig. 20 Normal fallopian tube and ovary as seen with laparoscopy.

3 / Childhood gynaecological disorders

Gynaecological disorders are uncommon in childhood.

Vulvovaginitis
This is the commonest gynaecological problem in children. There are three factors which make the immature vagina susceptible to infection:
- lack of protective acid secretion
- contamination by stool and debris
- impaired mechanisms of immunity.

The usual bacteriological finding is of mixed bacterial flora. The child will complain of vulval soreness, discharge, or pain on micturition. Threadworm infestation can sometimes cause this condition.

Foreign bodies
These usually produce a purulent discharge or bleeding.

Hydrocolpos
In this disorder, an imperforate membrane is situated immediately above the hymen. Above this obstruction the vagina can become distended by fluid (Fig. 21). Hydrocolpos can present in the neonate as retention of urine, abdominal pain and a lower abdominal swelling if there is a large quantity of fluid. The treatment is simple incision of the membrane to release the fluid.

Haematocolpos
The same situation as in hydrocolpos occurs in haematocolpos, except that the problem does not arise until puberty. The menstrual fluid is unable to be released and collects above the imperforate hymen, grossly expanding the vagina and even the uterus. The presenting symptoms may include abdominal pain, urinary retention or a large abdominal mass. Vulval inspection will reveal a bulging bluish membrane that requires incision.

Fused labia
Labial adhesions are not uncommon. The labia minora become adherent to each other (Fig. 22), and it may appear as though the vagina is absent. The aetiology is not known, but the condition is probably due to low oestrogen levels. Application of oestrogen cream usually results in spontaneous separation after 10–14 days.

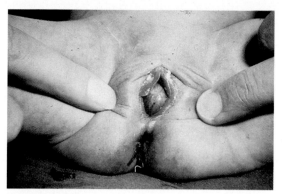

Fig. 21 Hydrocolpos.

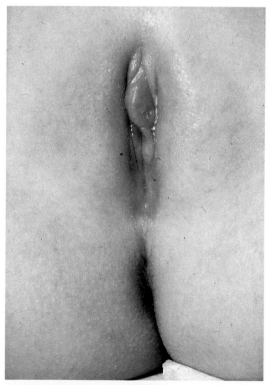

Fig. 22 Fused labia.

Botryoid sarcoma Tumours are rare in childhood, but embryonal rhabdomyosarcoma is the most serious. It is often grapelike in appearance (Fig. 23) but may appear simply as a polyp. The tumour spreads extensively in the subepithelial tissues of the vagina or ectocervix. Chemotherapy is generally given prior to extended hysterectomy or vaginectomy (Fig. 24).

Congenital abnormalities The Müllerian ducts are the embryological precursors of the fallopian tubes, uterus and upper two-thirds of the vagina. The lower one-third of the vagina develops from the urogenital sinus. Various defects can occur during embryological development (Fig. 25). These include:

- failure of development, e.g. no paramesonephric duct
- failure of paramesonephric duct canalization
- failure of fusion of paramesonephric ducts
- failure of median septum loss (Fig. 26)
- failure of fundal dome development
- failure of fusion of paramesonephric ducts with urogenital sinus
- failure of transverse septum loss between paramesonephric system and urogenital sinus.

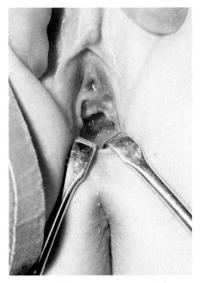

Fig. 23 Botryoid sarcoma at examination.

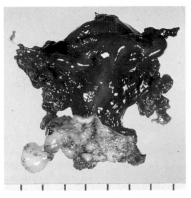

Fig. 24 Surgical specimen of botryoid sarcoma.

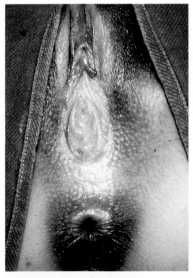

Fig. 25 Absent vagina — a congenital defect.

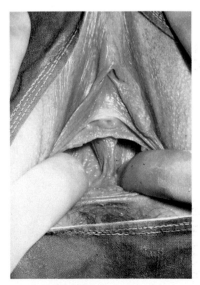

Fig. 26 Vaginal septum.

Sexual abuse

Children who have been sexually abused endure physical and psychological trauma. When sexual abuse is suspected, a thorough examination must be carried out by an experienced gynaecologist. Swabs for sexually transmitted diseases must be taken from the vagina, cervix and anus. Samples for semen should also be taken. Photographs should be taken if possible, and the signs of physical trauma accurately documented. The examinations are often performed under anaesthesia.

Vulval bruising is common, and the hymen is often perforated (Fig. 27). Anal bruising must be looked for (Fig. 28), and anal dilatation. The rest of the body must be searched for bruising or other signs of trauma. Fractures should be suspected. These children usually need admitting until the domestic situation has been thoroughly investigated.

Female circumcision

This barbaric custom is still practiced, mainly in Africa. The extent of the procedure varies. If performed early in infancy it is usually limited to trimming of the labia minora and tip of clitoris. Complications are rare. If the operation is carried out near puberty, haemorrhage and sepsis can be severe. Complete excision of the labia and minora is performed and the denuded edges are encouraged to unite by strapping the thighs together, with a stick between the edges to allow passage of urine. The resulting scarring can be extreme and the urethra and vestibule hidden (Fig. 29). This deflects the urinary stream causing chronic infection both of the surrounding skin and vagina. Intercourse may be impossible, and division of a skin bridge may be necessary. For vaginal delivery, an anterior episiotomy may be necessary. In obstructed labour, the fetus may be in the vagina for long enough to cause vaginal wall pressure necrosis.

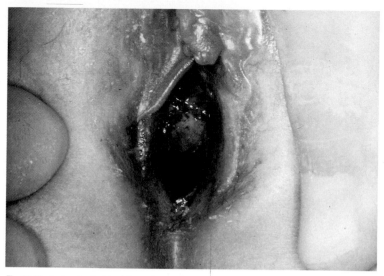

Fig. 27 Vaginal and vulval bruising.

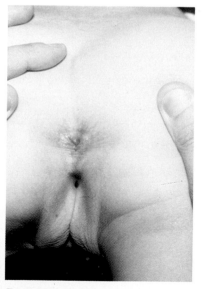

Fig. 28 Anal trauma.

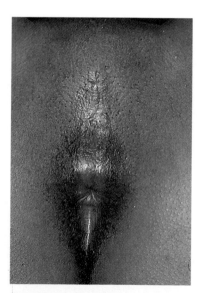

Fig. 29 Female circumcision.

Disorders of puberty

The hormonal changes of puberty are complex. Disordered function can reveal chromosomal, enzymatic and structural abnormalities not obvious in childhood.

Turner's syndrome

In Turner's syndrome (Fig. 30), the absence of the one sex chromosome leads to ovarian dysgenesis resulting in primary amenorrhoea, short structure and sexual infantilism. Alternatively, androgen-receptor defects with a normal XY complement lead to failure of masculinization and apparently normal, full breast development. Primary amenorrhoea may be the first presentation of this problem of testicular feminization (Fig. 31).

5 alpha reductase deficiency

In 5 alpha reductase deficiency (Fig. 32), the lack of the enzyme likewise results in failure of masculinization of the external genitalia in the genotypic male child. However, at puberty the large increase in testosterone production by normal, internalized testes results in androgenization of the presumed female. The testes are removed and oestrogen replacement ensures a phenotypic female.

Other problems include precocious puberty, as indicated by early thelarche or menarche, or delayed puberty where hypothalamic maturation is pathologically late.

Intersex

Definition

An intersex is an individual in whom there is discordance between chromosomal, gonadal, internal genital and phenotype sex, or the sex of rearing.

Clinical features

It may be declared at birth because of ambiguous external genitalia (Fig. 33), during childhood because of precocious puberty or during adolescence because pubertal changes are inappropriate to presumed gender, or because puberty fails to occur.

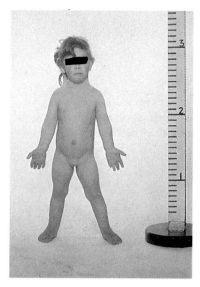

Fig. 30 Turner's syndrome.

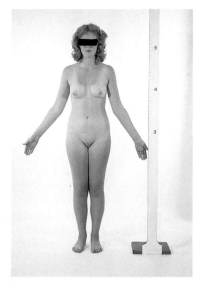

Fig. 31 Testicular feminization.

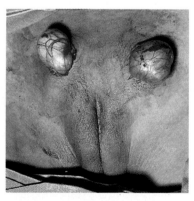

Fig. 32 Inguinal testes in 5 alpha reductase deficiency.

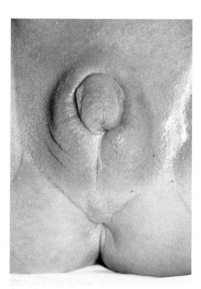

Fig. 33 Intersex.

4 / The menstrual cycle

Puberty At puberty the hypothalamic pituitary gonadal axis changes and gonadotrophin releasing hormone (GnRH) is secreted in a pulsatile fashion from the hypothalamus. This stimulates a pulsatile release of follicle-stimulating hormone (FSH) and luteinizing hormone (LH) from the anterior pituitary. Thereafter, FSH and LH are secreted in pulses every 70–220 minutes depending on the cycle phase. The release of the gonadotrophins is regulated by the ovarian steroid feedback on the hypothalamus and pituitary.

Hormonal changes At the beginning of each cycle (Fig. 34a), FSH stimulates growth in follicles, with one follicle becoming dominant while the others undergo atresia. Oestrogen production in the dominant follicle increases, leading to rising oestradiol blood levels. These high oestrogen levels trigger the LH surge from the pituitary which in turn causes ovulation. This LH surge also stimulates the production of progesterone and prostaglandins in the follicle. The oocyte is then released from the follicle which shrinks and then becomes the corpus luteum, which produces progesterone. Unless a pregnancy occurs, the corpus luteum will regress after about 10 days. If pregnancy does occur, the human chorionic gonadotrophin (HCG) maintains the production of steroids from the corpus luteum until the tenth week of pregnancy.

Endometrial changes The endometrium in the first half of the cycle (Fig. 34b) responds to the oestrogenic stimulation by growth of the glands and endometrial thickening. When progesterone is produced in the second half of the cycle, the epithelium lining the glands develops vacuoles, and the glands and the spiral arterioles continue to grow. The stroma becomes oedematous and undergoes decidualization.

Falling levels of oestrogen and progesterone cause cyclical constriction and dilatation of the spiral arterioles, and eventually generalized vasoconstriction, ischaemia and cell disintegration occur leading to release of lysosomal enzymes. Breakdown is halted by rising levels of oestrogen from the next follicle.

The cervix and vagina show dramatic changes in morphology and secretions in response to ovarian steroid output (Fig. 35, p. 26).

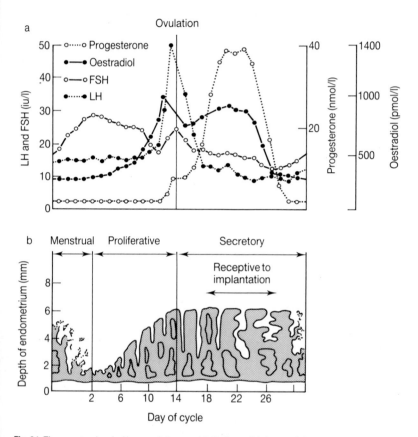

Fig. 34 The menstrual cycle. Hormonal changes (a). Endometrial changes (b).

Amenorrhoea

Amenorrhoea (failure to menstruate) can be due to
absence of the uterus (e.g. XY female), blockage of the
outflow tract due to imperforate hymen or endometrial
disturbances, i.e. absence as in intrauterine scarring
(Ascherman's syndrome), atrophy as in premature
menopause or hormonal imbalance as in polycystic
ovarian disease.

Primary Primary amenorrhoea has been mentioned in disorders of
puberty.

Secondary Secondary amenorrhoea is defined as the cessation of
periods for greater than six months. The commonest
pathological causes are hypothalamic suppression,
hyperprolactinaemia (usually due to prolactinoma, Fig.
36) or polycystic ovarian disease. Other causes include
thyroid disease, adrenal disease, premature ovarian failure
and Sheehan's syndrome. Obviously, pregnancy and
normal menopause are physiological causes.

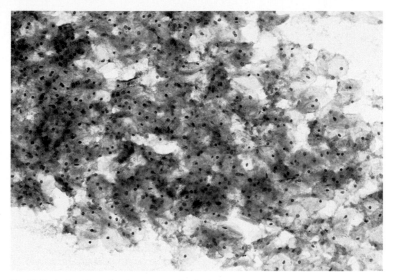

Fig. 35 Vaginal cytology showing oestrogenic stimulation.

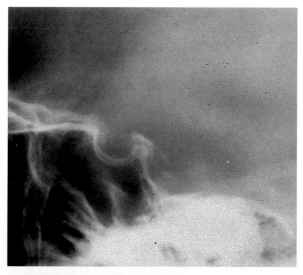

Fig. 36 Skull X-ray of enlarged pituitary fossa.

Dysfunctional uterine bleeding

Definition   Abnormal uterine bleeding after pelvic pathology has been excluded.

Aetiology   Not known.

Classification   Cases can be divided into anovulatory or ovulatory.

Clinical features   The majority of patients will report heavy bleeding which may be regular or irregular. It is extremely difficult to make an accurate assessment of the amount of bleeding by relying on history alone. Quantitative measurement of blood loss can be made by collecting all the tampons and sanitary pads and using the alkalin haematin test.

On abdominal and pelvic examination there should be no abnormalities detected.

Investigations   To exclude pelvic pathology, a thorough pelvic assessment must be made including cervical smear and endometrial biopsy if indicated (Figs 37 & 38). Ultrasound, laparoscopy, hysteroscopy or colour doppler studies are investigations that may be used depending on the clinical situation.

Management   ***Anovulatory***. In adolescents the oral contraceptive pill will make the withdrawal bleeds lighter, regular and less painful. In the perimenopausal woman, hormone replacement therapy or cyclical progestagens (after exclusion of uterine pathology) would be appropriate.

Ovulatory. Nonsteroidal anti-inflammatory drugs, the oral contraceptive pill, danazol and antifibrinolytic drugs are the main options.

Hysterectomy or endometrial ablation are used if the above measures fail.

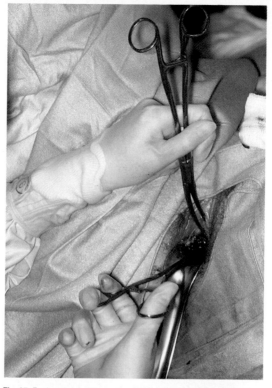

Fig. 37 Explorations of the endometrial cavity for polyps.

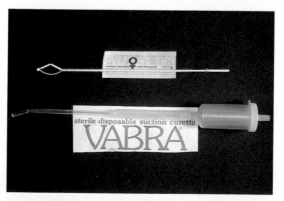

Fig. 38 Outpatient endometrial samplers.

5 / Contraception

A woman is at her most fertile at the time of ovulation, which in a 28-day cycle will occur about 14 days after the last menstrual period. Sperm may survive in the genital tract for up to 7 days, therefore, to avoid conception, intercourse should be discontinued one week before ovulation is expected and recommenced not less than 2 days after ovulation has occurred. Ovulation may be predicted by:

- monitoring previous cycles (rhythm method)
- using the rise in body temperature associated with ovulation to determine the 'safe period' (Fig. 39)
- assessing the texture of cervical mucus which becomes profuse and watery (spinbarkeit) at ovulation.

The failure rates for these methods may be as high as 25 pregnancies per hundred women years.

Coitus interruptus (removal of the penis from the vagina before ejaculation) is an old and widely used method of contraception. It is not particularly effective.

Barrier
methods
Condoms. When used in combination with a spermicide, e.g. Nonoxynol-9, condoms are a highly effective method of contraception, resulting in only 2 to 3 failures per hundred women years. Condoms also act as a physical barrier to the transmission of many sexually transmitted infections.

Caps. The diaphragm (Fig. 40) is the most commonly used; other types include cervical (Fig. 41) and vault caps. When used with spermicide, a diaphragm is as effective as a condom and spermicide. The diaphragm consists of a thin latex rubber dome attached to a circular metal spring. The size of the diaphragm required is determined during an examination by a family planning doctor. It should cover the cervix, with the anterior edge of the diaphragm lying behind the symphysis pubis, and the posterior edge lying comfortably in the posterior fornix. The diaphragm should be inserted prior to intercourse and should not be removed for at least six hours afterwards.

Others. Disposable sponges impregnated with Nonoxynol-9 are currently available, but they are expensive to buy and not very effective. A 'female condom' is currently under evaluation.

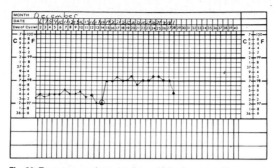

Fig. 39 Temperature chart—ovulatory biphasic pattern. Temperature rise follows ovulation and persists until just prior to menstruation.

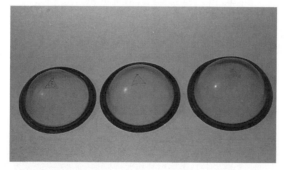

Fig. 40 Diaphragms.

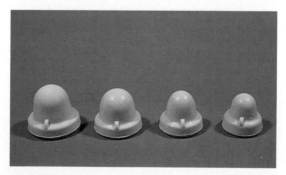

Fig. 41 Cervical caps.

Hormonal contraception

Combined oral contraceptive pills. These contain both oestrogen and progesterone (Fig. 42). They are taken cyclically for 21 days with a 7-day break. During the 'pill-free week,' a withdrawal bleed is experienced. The combined pill acts on the hypothalamus and pituitary causing inhibition of GnRH, FSH and LH by negative feedback, thus preventing ovulation. The endometrium is also rendered unsuitable for implantation. The progesterone element of the combined pill makes the cervical mucus impenetrable to sperm and may also interfere with fallopian tube function. The combined pill should not be used by women with hormone-dependent tumours (breast, endometrium, trophoblast). Thromboembolism, arterial disease, valvular heart disease, focal migraine, clotting abnormalities and liver disease are all contraindications to pill usage. Smoking, hypertension, and diabetes are considered 'relative contraindications'. The combined pill is the most effective reversible method of contraception currently available.

Progesterone only pills. These do not necessarily inhibit ovulation; they act on the endometrium, the endocervical mucus and the fallopian tubes. Progesterone only preparations (Fig. 43) should be taken at the same time every day, without any breaks. The maximal effect on cervical mucus is seen 4 to 6 hours after taking the pills. Even with good compliance, progesterone only pills are less effective than combined pills.

Depot progestogen injections. Used in sufficiently high doses, these will:

- inhibit ovulation
- render the endometrium atrophic
- thicken the cervical mucus.

This form of contraception is effective, safe, convenient and reversible. Some women will, however, suffer from weight gain and bleeding irregularities. Depo-Provera and Noristerat are the two depot injections marketed in the UK. Depo-Provera is given as one injection (150 mg) every twelve weeks. Noristerat is given 8-weekly (100 mg).

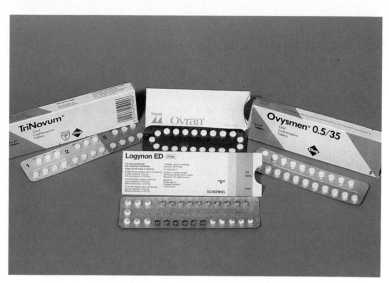

Fig. 42 Combined oral contraceptive pills.

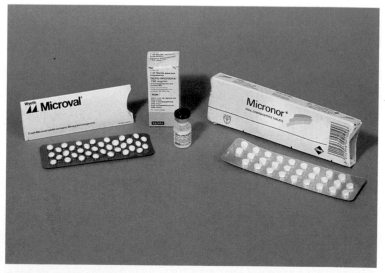

Fig. 43 Progestogen preparations.

Hormonal contraception (cont)

Postcoital contraception. Two combined oral contraceptive pills containing 50 μg of oestrogen are taken followed by a further two tablets 12 hours later. They must be taken within 72 hours of unprotected intercourse. This regimen causes nausea in up to 30% of takers. The overall failure rate is roughly 2%.

Intrauterine contraceptive devices (IUCD)

The IUCD (Fig. 44) is placed in the uterus by a doctor using a sterile technique. It acts by altering/inhibiting sperm migration and ovum transport. The sterile inflammatory response to the presence of a foreign body inhibits implantation of the blastocyst. It is a safe, highly effective and reversible form of contraception, but it must be fitted by a doctor and requires follow-up care. An intrauterine contraceptive device should not be fitted in women who have had pelvic inflammatory disease, or if there is an intrauterine pregnancy or uterine abnormality. It can be used as a method of postcoital contraception. To be effective it must be fitted within 5 days of unprotected intercourse.

Sterilization

Female methods of sterilization involve the blockage of the fallopian tubes. This can be achieved by excision or occlusion with clips (Fig. 45), rings, or by diathermy via the laparoscope or a mini-laparotomy. It is highly effective and should be considered irreversible. The failure rate is about 0.1%.

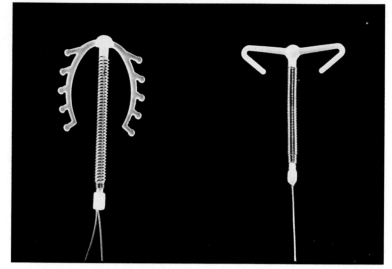

Fig. 44 Intrauterine contraceptive devices.

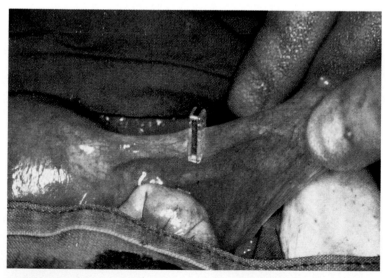

Fig. 45 Sterilization clip.

6 / Early pregnancy problems

Miscarriage

Definition   A spontaneous loss of pregnancy before 28 weeks.

Incidence   15 to 25% of all pregnancies end in miscarriage.

Classification   Miscarriage can be classified as follows (Fig. 46):

- *Threatened abortion:* fetus is still viable, and the cervical os is closed.
- *Inevitable abortion:* fetus may still be alive but the cervical os is open.
- *Incomplete abortion:* some products of conception have been expelled already.
- *Complete abortion:* fetus and placental tissue have all been expelled.
- *Missed abortion:* the pregnancy has succumbed but has not been expelled (Fig. 47, p. 38).

Aetiology   The majority of miscarriages are due to chromosomal defects. If they are in the first trimester it is not worth investigating women who miscarry—unless they have had three consecutive spontaneous miscarriages. The causes can be:

- abnormal conceptus (chromosomal or structural)
- immunological
- uterine abnormality
- cervical incompetence
- endocrine
- maternal disease (including systemic lupus erythematosus)
- infection
- toxins (e.g. cytotoxics)
- trauma.

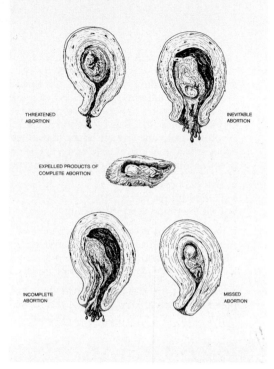

THREATENED
ABORTION

INEVITABLE
ABORTION

EXPELLED PRODUCTS OF
COMPLETE ABORTION

INCOMPLETE
ABORTION

MISSED
ABORTION

Fig. 46 Diagrammatic representation of types of miscarriage.

Clinical features
of miscarriage

Patients will present with amenorrhoea followed by vaginal bleeding. Pain may be present. The symptoms of pregnancy may have disappeared. On examination there may be lower abdominal tenderness. The bleeding may vary from spotting to heavy bleeding. The uterine size may be smaller than dates (if products have been expelled), the same size, or larger than dates (if bleeding has occurred into the uterine cavity). The cervix may be closed or open depending on the stage of the miscarriage.

Differential
diagnosis

- Ectopic pregnancy.
- Hydatidiform mole.
- Dysfunctional uterine bleeding.

Investigation

If the cervical os is open, the pregnancy will not continue and no further investigations are needed. If the os is closed, an ultrasound scan will determine whether a viable fetus is present in the uterine cavity (Fig. 47).

Management

There is no proven treatment for a threatened abortion. Inevitable, incomplete, complete and missed abortions all require evacuation of the uterus (Fig. 48).

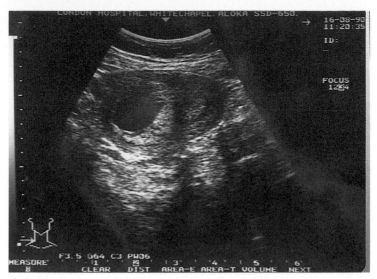

Fig. 47 Ultrasound picture of a blighted ovum in a bicornuate uterus.

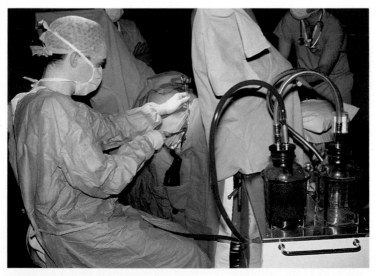

Fig. 48 Surgical evacuation of the uterus.

Ectopic pregnancy

Definition The implantation of a pregnancy outside the uterine cavity (usually in the ampullary part of the fallopian tube).

Aetiology Any factor that will decrease embryo transport along the tube can lead to an ectopic pregnancy. The most common cause is previous pelvic infection.

Pathophysiology The fertilized ovum is delayed in its transport along the tube and implants on the tubal mucosa. Intratubal or intraperitoneal bleeding occurs as a result of erosion and distension of the tubal wall (Fig. 49). The uterine endometrium undergoes decidualization in response to the hormonal stimulus of the trophoblast.

Symptoms Classically, the patient will have had amenorrhoea followed by irregular spotting or vaginal bleeding and unilateral pain (may be bilateral).

Signs These will vary depending on whether tubal rupture has occurred. If tubal rupture has occurred the patient may be in shock.

    The abdominal signs can vary from unilateral lower abdominal tenderness with rebound to a rigid abdomen with guarding. Vaginally there is usually cervical excitation and unilateral tenderness, and a mass may be felt on one side.

Differential diagnosis
● Miscarriage
● Pelvic infection

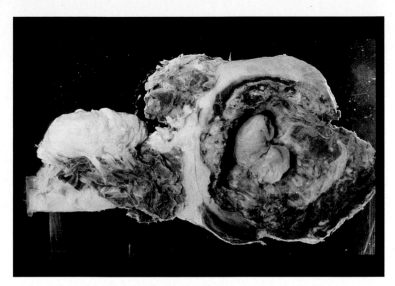

Fig. 49 Ectopic gestation distending the fallopian tube.

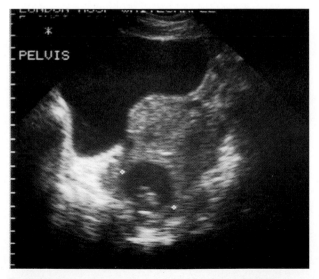

Fig. 50 Gestation sac lateral to the uterus which is indenting the bladder.

Investigations for ectopic pregnancy

Pregnancy test: should be positive if modern HCG assay is used.

Ultrasound scan: may be useful if an intrauterine pregnancy is demonstrated. Occasionally the ectopic pregnancy can be seen outside the uterine cavity (Fig. 50, p. 40), and free fluid can be seen in the Pouch of Douglas.

Blood sampling: for FBC and cross-matching.

Laparoscopy: should be performed if there is any suspicion of an ectopic pregnancy. The tube may be distended or filled with blood (Fig. 51). Some units are operating on ectopics with endoscopic surgical techniques.

Laparotomy: when there is no doubt as to the diagnosis, or when the diagnosis has been confirmed by laparoscopy.

Treatment

Resuscitation if needed. Surgery should be conservative. An attempt should be made to 'milk' the ectopic out of the tube. If this is not successful, a partial salpingectomy is performed or, rarely, a total salpingectomy.
Occasionally a tubal abortion may have occurred and the fetus may be free in the peritoneal cavity (Fig. 52).

Prognosis

Only one-third of women will proceed to have a successful term baby. About 10% will have a further ectopic.

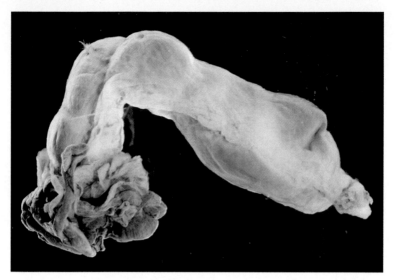

Fig. 51 Fallopian tube distended with blood.

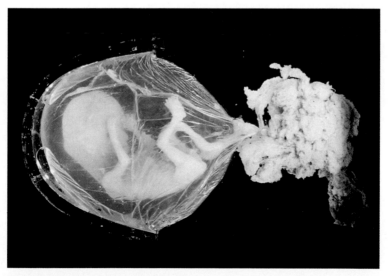

Fig. 52 Fetus found free in the peritoneal cavity.

Trophoblastic disease

Definition Hydatidiform mole is a benign tumour of trophoblast.

Incidence Varies geographically, with a higher incidence in Asiatic countries than in the West.

Aetiology Unknown.

Classification **Complete mole:** no fetus is present and the chromosomal complement is totally paternal. There are 46 chromosomes.
Partial mole: fetus is present. There are 69 chromosomes and the extra set is of paternal origin.
Invasive mole: may penetrate the uterus and/or metastasize to the lungs.

Clinical features The symptoms are usually irregular bleeding in the first trimester of pregnancy. The uterus may be larger than dates and the fetal heart is usually absent. Preeclampsia may develop early, and theca lutein cysts may be palpable.

Investigations Ultrasound will demonstrate a 'snowstorm' appearance, and the fetus will not be seen (Fig. 53). Beta HCG level is very high. A chest X-ray should be done to exclude pulmonary metastases.

Management Suction evacuation of the hydropic vesicles (Fig. 54). If uterine size is too large, extra-amniotic prostaglandins are used. Hysterectomy may be done in the older woman. It is essential to follow all women to ensure that the Beta HCG levels disappear. Pregnancy should be discouraged for at least 12 months.

Prognosis One in thirty moles develops into choriocarcinoma—a malignant tumour of trophoblastic tissue. Chemotherapy is the mainstay of treatment and close follow-up is essential.

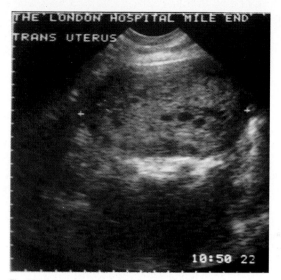

Fig. 53 Ultrasound picture of hydatidiform mole.

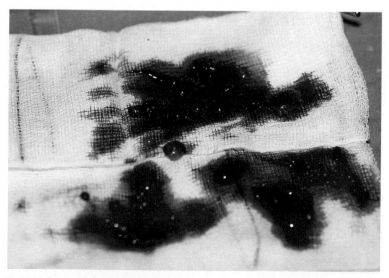

Fig. 54 Hydropic vesicles of hydatidiform mole.

7 / **Therapeutic abortion**

Definition   Medical termination of pregnancy prior to 24 weeks gestation.

Classification   Terminations can be performed for fetal or maternal reasons. Most are performed because the continuation of the pregnancy will cause risk to the physical or mental health of the woman.

Investigations   If gestation is in doubt, an ultrasound scan should be performed. Full blood count, blood group, rhesus status and haemoglobin electrophoresis should be undertaken if indicated.

Management   Counselling is essential in pregnancy termination. The appropriate forms must be filled out with two certifying practitioners. The method of termination will depend on the gestation.

RU486. This is a new progesterone antagonist which is used in combination with a prostaglandin pessary prior to 9 weeks gestation.

Dilatation and evacuation. The cervix is dilated (this can be made easier if a prostaglandin pessary is used prior to surgery) and then the uterine contents are removed, usually with a suction curettage (up to 14 weeks gestation; Fig. 55).

Prostaglandins. Labour is induced with prostaglandins after 14 weeks gestation. They can be administered as vaginal pessaries, intra-amniotically or extra-amniotically (Fig. 56). Whatever route, the procedure is followed by an evacuation of the uterus to ensure that the uterine cavity is empty.

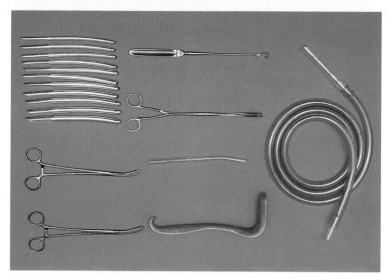

Fig. 55 Instruments used for suction termination of pregnancy.

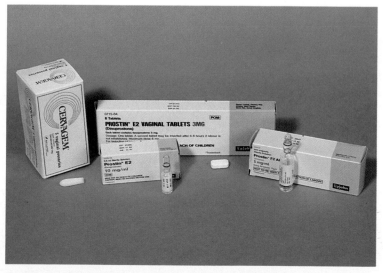

Fig. 56 Prostaglandin preparations used for the termination of pregnancy.

8 / Gynaecological infections

Lower genital tract infections

Vaginal discharge and vulvovaginitis are the most common manifestations of lower genital tract infection.

Candida (thrush)

Aetiology   Most cases are due to *Candida albicans* (a yeast like fungus). Yeasts may be present in the vagina without causing symptoms. Candida is not necessarily sexually transmitted, it can spread from the anus to the vulva and vagina. Once established, however, it can be transmitted sexually even by an asymptomatic partner.

Clinical features   Yeasts are the most common cause of vaginitis and vaginal discharge. The discharge is characteristically white, particulate, non-offensive and irritant. The vulva may appear red and oedematous and/or covered in white discharge (Fig. 57). In the vagina, white discharge (the texture of cottage cheese) adheres to the vaginal walls (Fig. 58). Yeasts can be identified by microscopy and Gram staining of a high vaginal swab, and by culture in the appropriate medium.

Management   Treatment includes topical antifungal agents, pessaries and creams, e.g. Clotrimazole and Nystatin. Severe cases or those resistant to local treatment may require systemic therapy with the newer oral antifungal agents such as fluconazole or ictaconazole.

Trichomonas vaginalis (TV)

Aetiology   TV is a flagellate parasite found in the vagina, the urethra (of both men and women) and in the upper genital tract. It is the second most common cause of vaginal discharge after candida. It is sexually acquired and is often found in association with gonorrhoea. The vaginal discharge is thin, yellow, offensive and irritant, often appearing frothy and causing reddening of the vaginal mucosa and the cervix (Fig. 59, p. 50). The organism is identified by microscopy of a high vaginal sample mixed with a drop of saline.

Management   Treatment involves metronidazole for both partners after screening for other sexually transmitted infections.

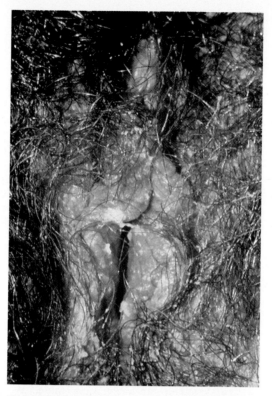

Fig. 57 Vulval candidiasis.

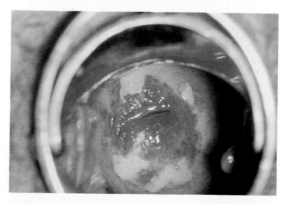

Fig. 58 Vaginal candidiasis.

Bacterial vaginosis

This is characterized by an offensive vaginal discharge which gives a positive amine test, has a pH greater than 5, and 'clue cells' seen on microscopy of a Gram stained smear. The cause is a mixed infection with *Gardnerella vaginalis* and anaerobic organisms including *Bacteroides* species and *Peptostreptococci*.

Other causes of vaginal discharge include increased but normal vaginal secretion, e.g. at ovulation, during sexual excitement or during pregnancy, and abnormal discharge due to chemical irritants, foreign bodies or degenerative conditions.

Warts (human papilloma virus; HPV)

Description Warts are caused by the human papilloma virus. They can be flat and undetectable to the naked eye, or large exophytic lesions. The cervix (Fig. 60), vaginal and vulval surfaces (Fig. 61) are all susceptible to infection. HPV has been strongly implicated as a causative factor in cervical neoplasia. The incubation period varies from 3 weeks to 8 months. It may present as painless slow growing vulvo-vaginal lumps. The differential diagnoses include molluscum contagiosum (caused by a pox virus) condylomata lata (lesions of secondary syphylis) and other skin tags, naevi or sebaceous cysts.

Management The following treatments are available: podophyllin (a cytotoxic agent), trichloracetic acid, electrocautery, cryocautery and excision. The last three are reserved for resistant and extensive warts.

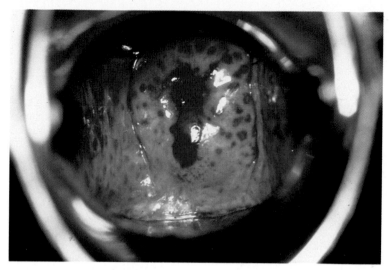

Fig. 59 Trichomonal 'strawberry cervix'.

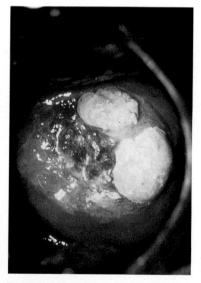

Fig. 60 Cervical warts.

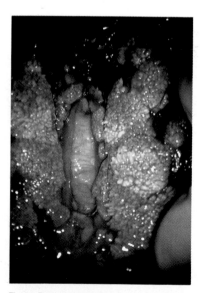

Fig. 61 Florid vulval warts.

Herpes simplex virus (HSV)

Aetiology   Genital and anal herpes are usually caused by type II HSV, but type I HSV (usually responsible for oral cold sores) can also be a cause of genital infection. In the UK, genital HSV is the most common identifiable cause of genital ulceration.

Clinical features   A primary infection may present with prodromal discomfort, followed by the appearance of vesicles (Fig. 62), ulceration, inguinal lymphadenopathy together with malaise, fever and possibly urinary retention. In women the vesicles are usually situated on the vulva (Fig. 63), vagina and cervix. The lesions of a primary infection may take several weeks to heal and secondary infection is common. Recurrence of HSV infection is common, as the virus lies dormant in the posterior nerve root ganglia between recurrences. Recurrent infection is less florid. Diagnosis is made on clinical examination and confirmed by viral cultures from the ulcers.

Management   Acyclovir can be used to reduce symptoms and virus shedding times in a primary attack. It does not prevent recurrences except during continuous treatment.

Complications   Primary infection can give rise to systemic complications, including hepatitis, myelitis, encephalitis and meningitis. A primary infection in early pregnancy may cause abortion. Infection near term may be transmitted to the baby during delivery leading to a high mortality rate and a high rate of neurological complications in the survivors. Primary infection or active recurrent disease at term are indications for delivery by ceasarean section before rupture of the membranes.

Other pathogens

Chlamydia trachomatis and *Neisseria gonorrhoeae* infect the cervix and urethra. They are usually asymptomatic in the absence of spread to the upper genital tract.

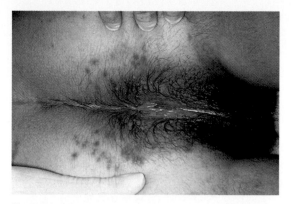

Fig. 62 Primary genital herpes infection.

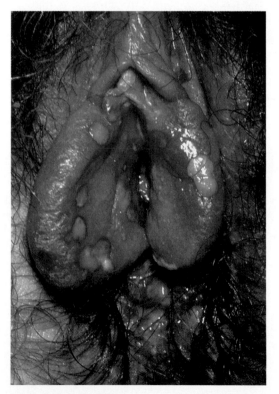

Fig. 63 Vulval herpes infection.

Pelvic inflammatory disease

Definition An infection of the endometrium, fallopian tubes and/or contiguous structures caused by the ascent of microorganisms from the lower genital tract.

Incidence Roughly 100 000 women in the UK develop PID each year. Most are women less than 25 years of age.

Aetiology The majority of cases of PID in young women are associated with sexually transmitted bacteria, e.g. *Chlamydia trachomatis* and *Neisseria gonorrhoeae*. These bacteria may initiate the process and then be replaced by opportunistic bacteria including streptococci and bacteroides.

Clinical features There is a spectrum of presentation from silent infection to florid symptoms and signs, i.e. pelvic pain, dyspareunia, fever, vaginal discharge, pyrexia, pelvic peritonism, cervical excitation and, possibly, a pelvic mass. Right upper quadrant pain may be due to perihepatitis (Fig. 64). It complicates up to 15% of cases of chlamydial PID. Laparoscopic evidence of PID (Fig. 65) is seen in only 65% of suspected cases.

Differential diagnoses These include acute appendicitis, endometriosis, ectopic pregnancy, ovarian cyst accident and inflammatory bowel conditions.

Management A combination of antibiotics active against all likely causative organisms, along with adequate analgesia, are required. In severe cases, hospital admission may be necessary. Surgery is appropriate if the condition fails to improve or deteriorates with conservative management. All women with PID and their partners should be referred to a genitourinary medicine clinic, screened for sexually transmitted infections and treated appropriately to avoid reinfection.

Complications Infertility follows in 15–20% of cases. There is a 7–10 fold increased risk of an ectopic pregnancy, and chronic pelvic pain is suffered by roughly 20% of women after PID.

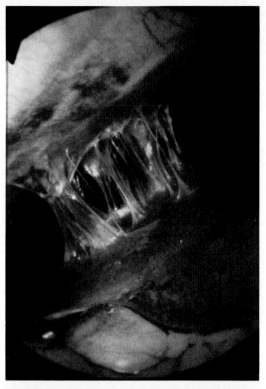

Fig. 64 Perihepatic adhesions (Fitz-Hugh–Curtis syndrome).

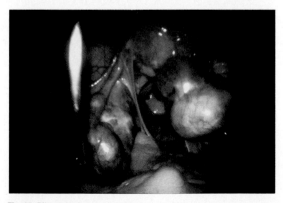

Fig. 65 Bilateral tubo-ovarian abscesses in PID.

HIV infection

Incidence and aetiology

HIV (human immunodeficiency virus) is most prevalent in Northern and Southern America, Sub-Saharan Africa and Western Europe. The age and sex distribution varies widely.

Mode of transmission

Sexual. Heterosexual intercourse is the most common mode of transmission/acquisition world wide. In Europe and North America, women are accounting for an increasing proportion of new cases.

Parenteral. Spread is from blood and blood products, before screening and heat treatment were introduced in 1985, and from sharing infected needles.

Transmission from mother to fetus. From 11 to 30% of children born to HIV antibody positive women will be infected (i.e. have antibodies persisting for greater than 18 months or develop clinical and or immunological manifestations of HIV at an earlier stage). Maternal health is an important factor in transmission of infection to the fetus. Of those infants who acquire HIV from their mothers, about 25% will develop AIDS in the first year of life.

Clinical features

AIDS is defined as an illness caused by HIV and characterized by one or more 'indicator' diseases which include candidiasis of the gastrointestinal (Fig. 66) and respiratory tract, cryptosporidiosis, *Pneumocystis carinii* pneumonia (Fig. 67) and toxoplasmosis of the brain (Fig. 68). Kaposi's sarcoma is rare in women; otherwise the spectrum of disease seen in men and women is similar.

Women and HIV

Important issues for women with HIV concern choice of contraception and wishes regarding pregnancy. There is no evidence that pregnancy accelerates the progress to AIDS. It has been suggested that the combined oral contraceptive pill may increase the risk of transmission and that an IUCD may put women with HIV at increased risk of pelvic inflammatory disease.

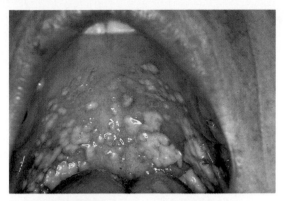

Fig. 66 Oral candidiasis.

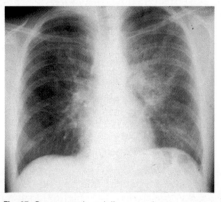

Fig. 67 *Pneumocystis carinii* pneumonia.

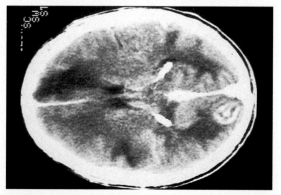

Fig. 68 Cerebral toxoplasmosis.

9 / Endometriosis

Definition   Endometriosis is a benign process characterized by the presence and proliferation of endometrial tissue in sites outside the uterine cavity.

Incidence   It is seen in up to 10% of premenopausal caucasian women and 30% of women presenting with infertility. The use of the oral contraceptive pill reduces the incidence of endometriosis.

Aetiology   A number of theories regarding the pathogenesis of endometriosis exist, but no single theory will explain all cases. The condition may therefore result from a combination of the following:

- *Retrograde menstruation:* the passage of endometrial tissue along the fallopian tubes during menstruation with implantation in the peritoneal cavity.
- *Lymphatic or vascular spread:* endometrial tissue embolizing to distant sites.
- *Metaplasia of coelomic epithelium:* the repeated inflammatory insult from menstrual blood in the peritoneal cavity may lead to redifferentiation of the peritoneal tissue and the development of viable endometrial tissue.

Pathology   A non-infectious process of inflammation, fibrosis and adhesion formation. The gross appearance is of black spots ('powder burns') (Fig. 69), commonly on the ovaries, uterosacral ligaments (Fig. 70) and Pouch of Douglas. Adhesion formation and distortion of normal anatomy may be a feature in severe disease (Fig. 71). If the ovaries are involved, 'chocolate cysts' may form. Unusual sites for endometriosis include the umbilicus, laparotomy scars, episiotomy scars, cervix (Fig. 72, p. 60), bowel, bladder, lung, thigh and vulva.

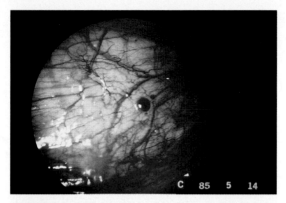

Fig. 69 Endometriotic deposit.

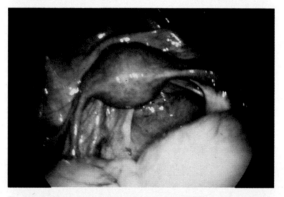

Fig. 70 Laparoscopy showing minimal endometriosis on left.

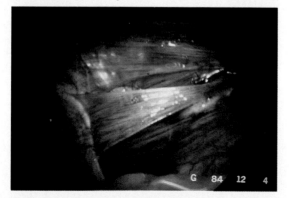

Fig. 71 Adhesions secondary to endometriosis.

Clinical features   These include pain, which may be cyclical, dypareunia, backache and secondary dysmenorrhea. Rarely there may be haematuria or rectal bleeding if the bladder or bowel are involved. Endometriosis may also be symptomless.

Investigations   The definitive diagnosis is made by laparoscopy or laparotomy. If haematuria or rectal bleeding are features, cystoscopy, sigmoidoscopy and barium enema would be necessary.

Management   Symptomatic disease can be treated medically or surgically.

Medical treatment
Medical treatment is based on the observation that endometriosis improves in pregnancy. The use of the oral contraceptive pill, without breaks for withdrawal bleeds, for up to nine months mimics pregnancy and is associated with symptomatic improvement. Progestagens, e.g. medroxyprogesterone acetate, also suppress ovulation and give relief from symptoms. Danazol (a testosterone derivative) is the most commonly used treatment. It creates a high androgen/low oestrogen environment which does not support the growth of endometrium. LHRH analogues given intranasally (Fig. 73) or subcutaneously suppress ovulation at the hypothalamus. They are as effective as Danazol and medroxyprogesterone acetate but are expensive, and the long-term effects of the low level of oestrogens on bone are not certain.

Surgical treatment
Surgical approaches can be through the laparoscope (diathermy or laser ablation and division of adhesions) or by laparotomy to restore pelvic anatomy or remove the uterus and ovaries.

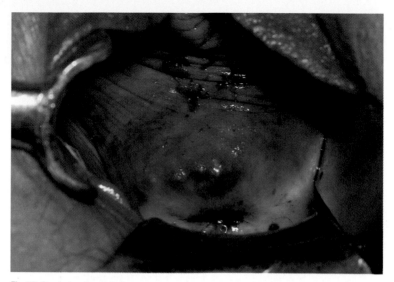

Fig. 72 Cervical endometriosis.

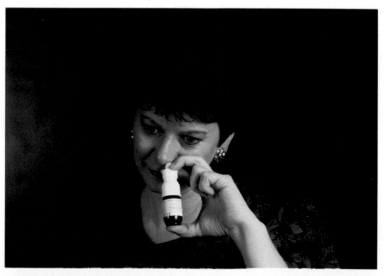

Fig. 73 LHRH analogue administered intranasally.

10 / Infertility

Definition   Infertility is defined as the failure to conceive after 12 months of regular unprotected intercourse. One out of six couples are affected.

Classification   **Primary:** no previous pregnancies.
Secondary: previous pregnancies.

Aetiology   The three main causes of infertility are poor semen quality, tubal disorders and ovulatory disorders. In addition, other rarer causes include mucus 'hostility' and sperm antibodies, impotence and retrograde ejaculation. This leaves a significant (10–20%) proportion with unexplained infertility which includes psychological factors.

Clinical features   Significant clues to the aetiology of the infertility can be achieved by a thorough history from both partners. In the female, evidence of ovulation can be gained from regularity of menstrual cycle and associated symptoms, e.g. mittleschmerz pain, cervical mucus changes and primary dysmenorrhoea.

Tubal disorders are usually the result of scarring and adhesions secondary to infection (Figs 74 & 75) or pelvic surgery, e.g. ovarian cystectomy or appendectomy. In addition, endometriosis may cause pelvic scarring and adhesions. If the distal portion of the tube is blocked, a hydrosalpinx may develop (Fig. 76). Tubal damage should be suspected if there is a history of IUCD use, PID, pelvic surgery or pelvic pain.

Examination may also reveal endocrinological disorders, e.g. PCOS, or the tissue atrophy of premature menopause, and physical signs of pelvic pathology, e.g. endometriotic scarring, ovarian cysts or fibroids.

In the male, history may reveal previous operations or infections. Stress and recent intercurrent illnesses, e.g. severe viral infection may be associated with transitory reduced semen quality. Examination should include testicles, looking for varicosities or the absence of the vas deferens. Reduced testicular size and increased firmness due to fibrosis may indicate spermatogenic failure. A swollen epididymis may indicate a blockage of the vas.

Rarely, azoospermia may be due to hypogonadotrophic hypogonadism which is indicated by lack of secondary sexual development.

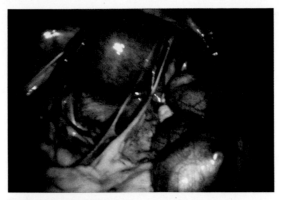

Fig. 74 Pelvic adhesions after PID.

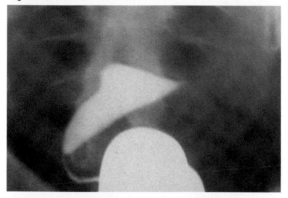

Fig. 75 Cornual blockage.

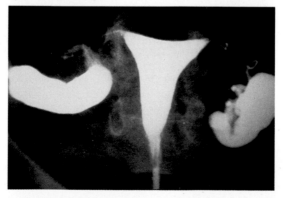

Fig. 76 Bilateral hydrosalpinges.

Differential diagnosis	Defining the specific causes of infertility requires a proper history and examination and appropriate investigations as outlined below.
Investigations	**Male** For the male, a semen analysis on two occasions is the basic investigation. The WHO criteria for a normal semen analysis is a sperm density of $\geq$ 20 million/ml with $\geq$ 50% motility and $\geq$ 50% normal sperm. The criteria are associated with a normal rate of conception. If the values are reduced, serum LH, FSH and testosterone are indicated. High gonadotrophins are indicative of failure. Normal levels with reduced testosterone may indicate hypogonadotrophic hypogonadism. There is rarely an indication for testicular biopsy.

Female

In the female, simple tests for ovulation should be undertaken, i.e. mid-luteal phase serum progesterone, basal body temperature charts (Fig. 77) for no more than 2 cycles. More sophisticated investigations include follicle monitoring with ultrasound (Fig. 78), serial LH measurements to detect the pre-ovulatory LH surge, and laparoscopy in the luteal phase to confirm the presence of a corpus luteum.

Laparoscopy and dye instillations (Fig. 79) provide the optimum test of tubal patency or damage with additional benefit of visualization of the pelvis, i.e. ovaries (for the presence of corpus luteum), peritoneum to exclude endometriotic deposits, and the uterus to assess anatomical abnormality. Hysterosalpingography is used to assess tubal patency and also to reveal intrauterine problems, e.g. adhesions, fibroids or anatomical abnormalities such as bicornuate uterus. (Fig. 80, p. 66). Other investigations include a post-coital test which assesses the capacity of sperm to remain motile in the cervical mucus, and tests for antisperm antibodies in both partners and in the husband's seminal plasma.

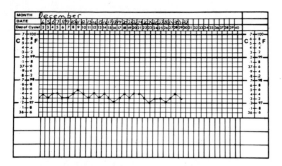

Fig. 77 Temperature chart showing an anovulatory pattern with absence of luteal phase rise.

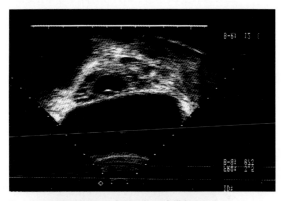

Fig. 78 Ultrasound image of a dominant follicle.

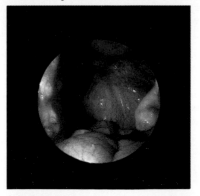

Fig. 79 Tubal patency as shown by presence of blue dye in the pelvis.

Management

Male

Poor semen quality has little opportunity for improvement unless it is a transitory problem, e.g. stress or viral infection. The value of varicocele repair is unresolved. Hormonal treatments are unproven. With low counts, options that are now available include the preparation of a small volume of the best sperm to place within the uterus at ovulation (intrauterine insemination; IUI) or in-vitro fertilization (IVF) with oocytes collected from the patient. Antisperm antibodies have been successfully treated with steroids in the male. Donor semen remains the only option for many infertile men.

Female

Ovulatory disorders respond well to hormonal therapy, i.e. clomiphene or human menopausal gonadotrophins. The latter requires close monitoring to avoid hyperstimulation or high-order multiple pregnancy. The damage can be dealt with by tubal surgery (Fig. 81) in selected cases, but the results rarely exceed 30%.

Bypassing the tube with IVF is successful in 15–20% of cycles. This involves ovarian stimulation to produce multiple follicles, the aspiration of the oocytes from these follicles, the in-vitro fertilization with partner's semen and transfer to the uterus 48 hours after fertilization.

Assisted conception techniques including IVF and gamete intrafallopian transfer (GIFT; Fig. 82) are also applicable where mucus hostility is a possible cause or where no cause is found, e.g. unexplained infertility. Success rates in these groups are between 25–30%.

Complications

The major complication of infertility other than those associated with drugs and surgical intervention is the psychological trauma of being unable to conceive. Significant morbidity is present in many couples who require counselling and support to enable them to come to terms with childlessness.

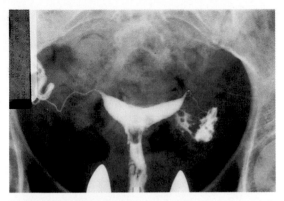

Fig. 80 Hysterosalpingogram of bicornuate uterus.

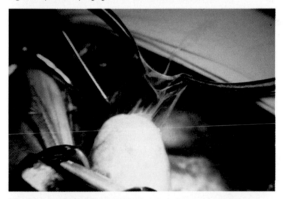

Fig. 81 Freeing of pelvic adhesions.

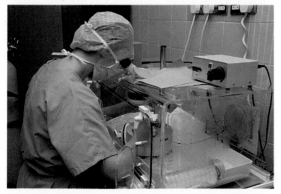

Fig. 82 Embryologist selecting oocytes during GIFT.

11 / Polycystic ovarian syndrome (PCOS)

Definition PCOS is a syndrome complex which involves oligoamenorrhoea, hirsutism (Figs 83 & 84), obesity and infertility; it is associated with disordered pituitary gonadotrophin secretion and ovarian steroid production.

Incidence Depending on the criteria used (clinical or ultrasound), the incidence varies from 5–30% of the female population. Amongst amenorrhoeic women, 30–40% probably have PCOS. Amongst hirsute women that incidence rises to 50–70%.

Aetiology The cause of PCOS is uncertain. There are two main hypotheses:
- ovarian enzyme abnormality resulting in abnormal steroid production
- disordered feedback mechanisms acting at the pituitary, resulting in abnormal gonadotrophin secretion with secondary ovarian dysfunction.

A small proportion of PCOS cases have been shown to be familial and due to ovarian enzyme abnormalities. The net result is an increased LH secretion, anovulation and increased ovarian androgen production.

Pathology The classical polycystic ovary is increased in size due to:
- increased stromal tissue
- multiple cystic ovaries, 2–4 mm in diameter, distributed around the periphery of the ovary (pearl nodi; Fig. 85 & Fig. 86, p. 70).

Clinical features Obesity is usually present from childhood, while hirsutism usually appears at puberty, affecting the face, chest and abdomen. Oligoamenorrhoea is present from puberty, often with episodes of secondary amenorrhoea. Infertility is usually primary.

Differential diagnosis Increased adrenal androgen production could also mean:
- Cushing syndrome
- adrenal hyperplasia
- adrenal carcinoma.

Hirsutism could also be familial, or due to drugs, while other causes of secondary amenorrhoea include hyperprolactinaemia. Other causes of infertility can be found on page 61.

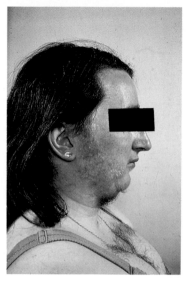

Fig. 83 Hirsutism before treatment.

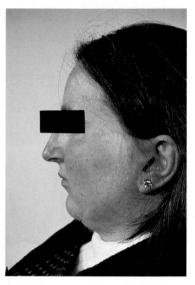

Fig. 84 Same patient in Figure 83 after hormone treatment.

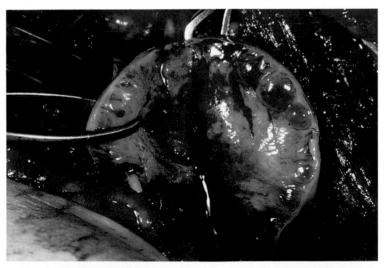

Fig. 85 Cut surface of polycystic ovary.

Investigations	**Biochemical:** serum LH, FSH, prolactin, testosterone (DHEAS, androstenedione).

Ultrasound: ovaries and pelvis (Fig. 87) (laparoscopy/ovarian biopsy).

Management   **Hirsutism:** management includes—

- cosmetic treatments (cream, waxing and electrolysis)
- oral contraceptive pill with low androgenic progestogen
- anti-androgens (cyproterone acetate (Fig. 84, p. 68) and spironolactone).

Obesity is treated with diet.

Oligoamenorrhoea/amenorrhoea: treatment includes—

- oral contraceptive pill to produce regular withdrawal bleeds
- clomiphene (will produce regular cycles in 50% but will also induce ovulation).

Infertility: induction of ovulation with clomiphene is successful in 70–80% of women with PCOS, with pregnancy rates equivalent to regularly ovulating women. If not successful, HMG, with or without pituitary down regulation using LHRH analogues, is usually effective. This latter regime can result in severe ovarian hyperstimulation. (Fig. 88).

Complications   This group of obese, anovulatory women are more likely to develop endometrial hyperplasia and adenocarcinoma in later life. Regular shedding of the endometrium induced by progestogens or OCP seems a logical, though unproven, prophylaxis.

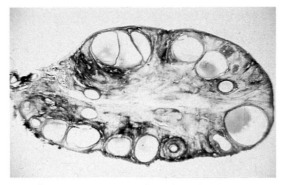

Fig. 86 Microscope section of polycystic ovary.

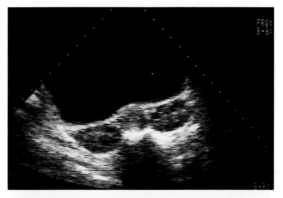

Fig. 87 Ultrasound showing polycystic ovaries.

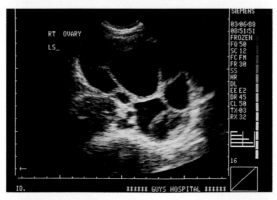

Fig. 88 Hyperstimulation in a polycystic ovary as seen by ultrasound.

12 / Benign and malignant conditions of the vulva and vagina

Pruritus vulvae

Aetiology   Vulval irritation can occur at any age, and the causes are numerous. The most common are infection, oestrogen deficiency and vulval dystrophies in the older woman.

Pathology   The commonest infective agent is candida. The dystrophies can be hypoplastic, hyperplastic or a mixed pattern. Paget's disease of the vulva usually presents in the elderly (Fig. 89). Vulval intraepithelial carcinoma (VIN) is a precursor to invasive carcinoma.

Clinical features   Irritation and itchiness of the vulva are present. On examination there may be evidence of excoriation, discolouration (Fig. 90), thickening or thinning of the vulval skin.

Bartholin's glands

These are paired structures which lie deep to the posterior introitus. They can become infected and present as a large tender swollen abscess. Marsupialization is the treatment of choice. Cyst formation can also occur.

Urethral caruncle

The external urethral meatus protrudes (Fig. 91) and swells. It may bleed, and may be very tender. Urethral caruncles are often associated with infection. If surgery is performed, the excised piece of tissue should be sent for histological confirmation to exclude urethral carcinoma.

Condylomata acuminata

Venereal warts are common on the vulva (Fig. 92) or in the vagina. They can be treated by topical applications, local destructive methods or surgery.

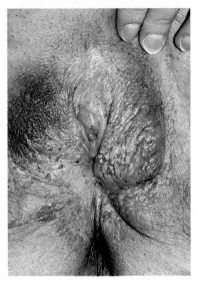

Fig. 89 Paget's disease of the vulva.

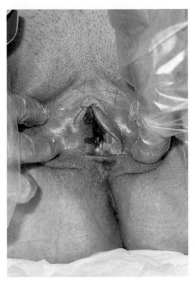

Fig. 90 Hypotrophic vulval dystrophy.

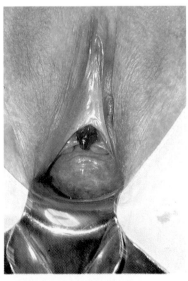

Fig. 91 Urethral caruncle with cystocoele.

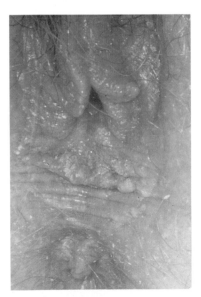

Fig. 92 Vulval warts.

Carcinoma of the vulva

Incidence Vulval carcinoma is an uncommon disease confined to elderly women.

Aetiology The vulva is an ideal site for skin irritation—warm and moist, prone to friction, poor hygiene and scratching.

Pathology Carcinoma of the vulva (Fig. 93) is usually a slow-growing and well-differentiated squamous carcinoma. Most of the lymphatics drain directly to the superficial and deep inguinal nodes, and then to the iliac chain.

Clinical features The woman usually presents with a history of chronic vulval irritation. She may have delayed seeking advice owing to embarrassment. The lesion is usually an epitheliomatous ulcer but sometimes may be in a 'cauliflower' form. The surrounding epithelium may show features of an underlying vulval dystrophy (Fig. 90, p. 72).

Management All suspicious lesions must be biopsied. If vulval intra-epithelial neoplasia (VIN) is diagnosed then simple vulvectomy is appropriate. Invasive carcinoma is best managed with a radical vulvectomy which consists of excision of the vulva with bilateral superficial and deep lymphadenectomy (Fig. 94 and Figs 95 & 96, p. 76).

Complications The morbidity and mortality from the operation are high, but the alternative is an unpleasant demise from a foul, fungating and painful growth.

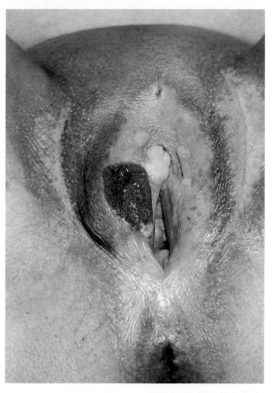

Fig. 93 Vulval carcinoma with surrounding intraepithelial neoplasia.

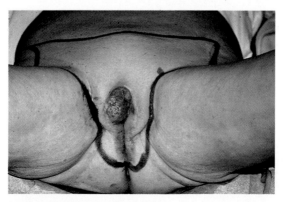

Fig. 94 Incision line for radical vulvectomy.

Carcinoma of the vagina

Incidence Carcinoma of the vagina is rare and occurs mainly in the sixth and seventh decades.

Classification The lesion may be primary (Fig. 97) or secondary, and is mainly squamous in origin. Staging is as follows:

Stage I—limited to vaginal wall
Stage II—involves subvaginal tissue
Stage III—extension to the pelvic wall
Stage IV—spread to adjacent or distant organs.

Clinical features Presenting symptoms are vaginal bleeding or a purulent discharge.

Investigations Biopsy must be performed.

Management Treatment of the condition is determined by histology, staging and health of the patient. Both surgery, radiotherapy and a combination of both have been used.

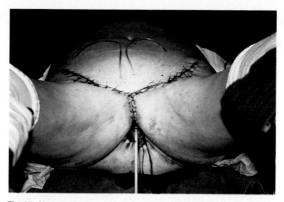

Fig. 95 Closure of skin incisions in radical vulvectomy.

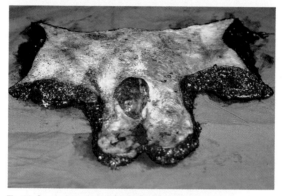

Fig. 96 Surgical specimen of vulval carcinoma.

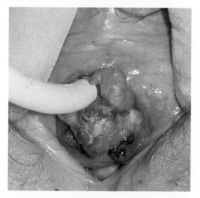

Fig. 97 Vaginal carcinoma.

13 / Benign, premalignant and malignant conditions of the cervix

The normal cervix

The normal ectocervix is covered with stratified squamous epithelium. The endocervical canal is lined by columnar epithelium. The junction between these two types is known as the *squamocolumnar junction*.

The position of the squamocolumnar junction varies. Puberty, pregnancy, and the use of the oral contraceptive pill cause eversion of the canal, thereby displaying a greater area of columnar epithelium which has a red appearance to the naked eye. This is termed *ectopy*. It is a normal physiological response, and the term erosion should not be used in this context. The area medial to the squamocolumnar junction is called the *transformation zone*.

Benign conditions

Cervicitis Certain bacteria preferentially infect columnar epithelium, e.g. *Chlamydia trachomatis* and *Neisseria gonorrhoeae*, giving rise to appearances described as cervicitis (Fig. 98).

Cervical fibroids These may be pedunculated or within the body of the cervix (Fig. 99), perhaps growing to a size that fills the vagina.

Cervical polyps These usually arise from the endocervix and are pedunculated with a covering of endocervical epithelium. They vary considerably in size and appear as bright red vascular growths (Fig. 100). Endocervical polyps may be symptomless or may present with irregular vaginal bleeding and/or postcoital bleeding. Treatment is by avulsion. If the base is broad it may require ligation.

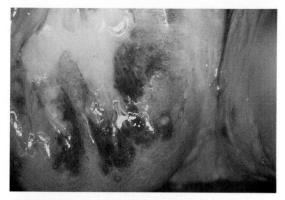

Fig. 98 Cervicitis.

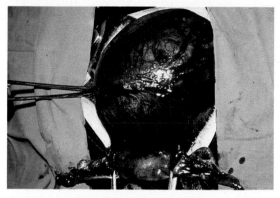

Fig. 99 Cervical fibroid at abdominal hysterectomy.

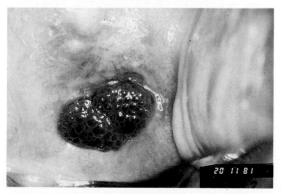

Fig. 100 Endocervical polyp. Colpophotograph.

Premalignant conditions

The transformation zone of the cervix normally undergoes metaplasia. However, it may, under certain circumstances also become dysplastic.

Clinical features Premalignant conditions of the cervix do not look abnormal to the naked eye. They are identified by cervical smear screening. The smear may demonstrate dyskaryotic cells (Fig. 101), graded as mild, moderate or severe (Fig. 102), depending on the degree of atypia. A dyskaryotic cell is clearly recognizable as a squamous cell but displays some of the features of malignancy; the nucleus is enlarged, the chromatin is increased and the nuclear borders are irregular.

Investigations Colposcopy is used to identify the lesion giving rise to the dyskaryotic cells exfoliated by the cervical smear. Using acetic acid to stain the cervix, areas of immature metaplasia (Fig. 103) and dysplasia (Fig. 104, p. 82) are seen as white ('acetowhite'). The density of this whiteness together with other features, including *punctation* (Fig. 105, p. 82), *mosaicism* (Fig. 106, p. 82), and *atypical vessel formation*, suggest the degree of abnormality present. Punch biopsies are taken from these abnormal areas to make a histological diagnosis.

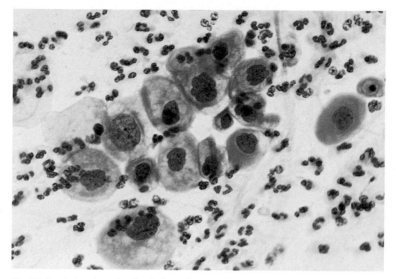

Fig. 101 Cervical cytology showing dyskaryosis.

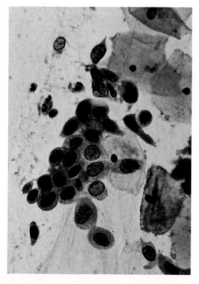

Fig. 102 Cervical cytology showing severe dyskaryosis.

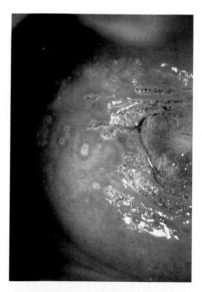

Fig. 103 Metaplasia colpophotograph.

Grading The histological findings are graded as CIN (cervical intraepithelial neoplasia) I, II and III, depending on the degree of dysplasia. Dysplasia is a histological term used to describe a lesion in which part of the thickness of the epithelium is replaced by atypical cells (Fig. 107, p. 84).

CIN I: the atypia is confined to the basal one-third of the epithelium.

CIN II: the basal two-thirds are involved and the changes are more marked.

CIN III (Figs 108 & 109, p. 84): nuclear abnormalities are present throughout the whole thickness of the epithelium.

If untreated, CIN may progress to cervical cancer.

Predisposing factors These include young age at first intercourse, sexual activity in women and their partners, prolonged use of the oral contraceptive and cigarette smoking.

Management Destruction of the whole transformation zone including all the areas of abnormal epithelium is undertaken using laser, cold coagulation, electrocautery, diathermy loop excision or cone biopsy. Cone biopsy is reserved for cases where colposcopic visualization of the transformation zone is incomplete. It is associated with risks of haemorrhage, cervical stenosis and cervical incompetence. Electrocautery and cone biopsy are performed under general anaesthetic, while all the others can be performed under local anaesthesia.

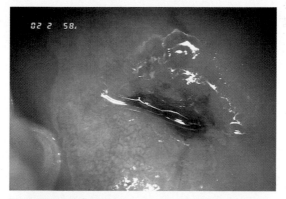

Fig. 104 Acetowhite changes.

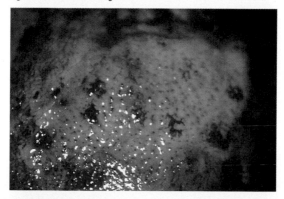

Fig. 105 Marked punctation.

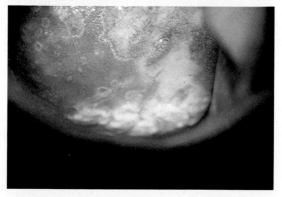

Fig. 106 Florid mosaicism.

Carcinoma of the cervix

Incidence Despite a screening programme aimed at the prevention of cervical cancer, the incidence is continuing to rise. There are approximately 4000 new cases reported each year in England and Wales. About 50% of these women will die from the disease within 5 years of diagnosis.

Staging Cancer of the cervix is staged clinically. An examination under anaesthesia is performed, combined with cervical biopsy, endometrial curettage and cystoscopy.

Stage I
- Ia Microinvasive disease. Lesions with a depth of invasion through the basement membrane of less than 5 mm and with a horizontal spread of less than 7 mm.
- Ib All other cases confined to the cervix (Fig. 110, p. 86).

Stage II
The carcinoma extends beyond the cervix but has not extended onto the pelvic sidewall. The carcinoma involves the vagina but not as far as the lower one-third.
- IIa No obvious parametrial involvement.
- IIb Obvious parametrial involvement.

Stage III
Carcinoma extends to the pelvic side wall. The lower one-third of the vagina may be involved. All cases with a hydronephrosis or a non-functioning kidney, unless they are known to be due to another cause.
- IIIa No extension onto the pelvic side wall, but involvement of the lower one-third of the vagina.
- IIIb Extension onto the pelvic side wall.

Stage IV
Carcinoma has extended beyond the true pelvis or has clinically involved the mucosa of the bladder or rectum.

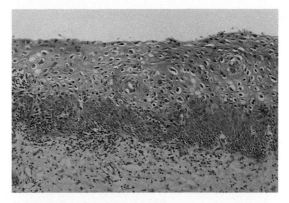

Fig. 107 Human papilloma virus and CIN.

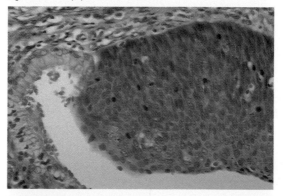

Fig. 108 CIN III and normal endocervix.

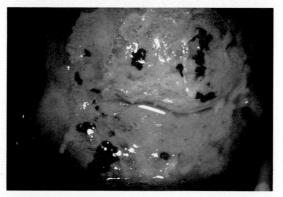

Fig. 109 Macroscopical view of CIN III.

Aetiology   Carcinoma of the cervix is more frequently seen in developing countries and its incidence is higher in lower socioeconomic groups. Cancer of the cervix is essentially a sexually transmitted disease. A number of factors transmitted during intercourse have been proposed; presently the wart virus has the strongest association. The risk of cervical cancer may be increased in long-term pill users and in women who smoke.

Pathology   Up to 90% of cervical cancers are squamous cell tumours originating in the transformation zone. Adenocarcinomas account for the remainder of cases. Cervical cancer spreads by direct extension or via the lymphatics.

Clinical features   Patients may present with vaginal bleeding, particularly after intercourse. There may be vaginal discharge. Early lesions may be symptomless and are detected by screening.

Investigations   Once the diagnosis is confirmed histologically (Fig. 111), an EUA is necessary for staging. Chest X-ray, IVP and routine biochemical and haematological investigations are usually required. CT scan is helpful in advanced and recurrent disease. Lymphangiography is performed by some to look for lymphatic spread.

Management   Hysterectomy is usually advised for microinvasive disease. Cone biopsy may be considered in a young woman desiring children. Stage Ib or IIa cervical cancer can be treated by either radiotherapy or Wertheim's hysterectomy (removal of the uterus, fallopian tubes, upper one-third of the vagina, parametrium and pelvic lymph nodes). Wertheim's hysterectomy is the treatment of choice in younger women who wish to retain ovarian function and avoid vaginal stenosis and gastrointestinal side effects which may be caused by radiotherapy. The results of radiotherapy and radical surgery in early stage disease are similar, both having 5 year survival rates in excess of 80%. The finding of tumour in lymph nodes will halve this survival rate. Radiotherapy is commonly used in more advanced disease. The role of chemotherapy is under evaluation.

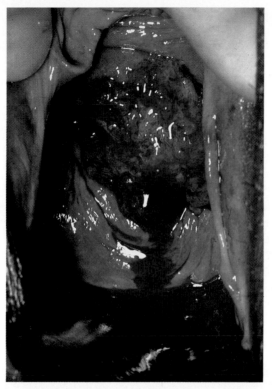

Fig. 110 Frank invasive carcinoma of the cervix.

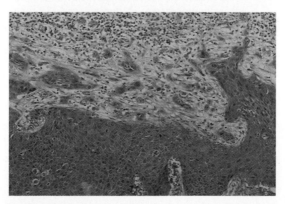

Fig. 111 Invasive squamous carcinoma.

14 / Benign and malignant conditions of the uterus

Congenital anomalies

Congenital absence of the uterus is rare, and in such cases a rudimentary vagina may be present. Congenital anomalies range from an arcuate uterus to a complete duplication of the uterus and cervix (see Figs 112, 113 & 114).

Fibroids

Definition   A common smooth muscle tumour also known as leiomyomata.

Incidence   Fibroids occur in more than 20% of caucasian women over 30 years.

Classification
- *Subserous:* project from the peritoneal surface of the uterus.
- *Intramural:* lie within the uterine wall.
- *Submucous:* encroach on the uterine cavity.
- *Pedunculated:* can arise from subserous or submucous.

Aetiology   Unknown.

Pathology   Fibroids arise from smooth muscle cells during reproductive life and can increase in size in response to oestrogen.

Clinical features   The majority of fibroids are symptomless. They may cause menorrhagia, abdominal distension and pressure symptoms such as urinary frequency. Pain is unusual unless there is red degeneration or torsion of a pedunculated fibroid.

Abdominal examination may reveal a palpable mass arising from the pelvis. Pelvic examination will confirm this and the outline may be irregular.

Differential diagnosis   Ovarian mass is the most common. It is often difficult to distinguish whether the pelvic mass is separate from the uterus.

Investigations   These include ultrasonography. EUA, hysteroscopy, dilatation and curettage if abnormal bleeding.

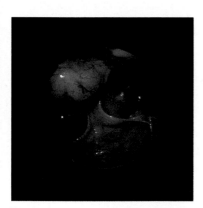

Fig. 112 Laparoscopic view of bicornuate uterus.

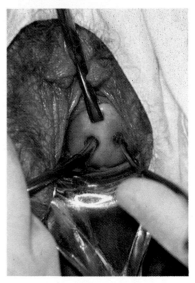

Fig. 113 A double cervix with a dilator in each os.

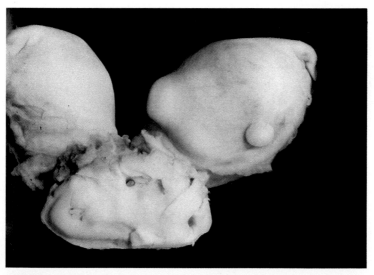

Fig. 114 Pathological specimen of uterus bicollis bicornuas.

Management of fibroids Treatment can either be conservative or surgical (Fig. 115). Factors determining management are: age, uterine size, presence of symptoms, fertility wishes and rate of growth.

Complications The poor vascularity of fibroids encourages the following changes: degeneration (hyaline, cystic, red, sarcomatous), calcification (Fig. 116) and/or necrosis. Fibroids can also become infected, tort and rarely metastasize.

Endometrial carcinoma

Classification The majority of lesions are adenocarcinoma (Fig. 117), and the staging is as follows:
Stage I—confined to the body of the uterus.
Stage II—involves the body and the cervix.
Stage III—extends beyond uterus but not beyond the true pelvis.
Stage IV—extends outside true pelvis or involves bladder or rectum.

Aetiology Endometrial carcinoma occurs in postmenopausal women and women who have had prolonged exposure to oestrogen stimulation, i.e. nulliparous women, late menopause, obese women and women with polycystic ovaries. Hyperplasia is a precursor.

Clinical features Classically, the postmenopausal women presents with bleeding. On examination the uterus may be normal sized or enlarged.

Clinical features The presenting symptoms are vaginal bleeding or a purulent discharge.

Investigations Biopsy must be performed.

Management Treatment is determined by histology, staging and health of the patient. Both surgery, radiotherapy and a combination of both have been used.

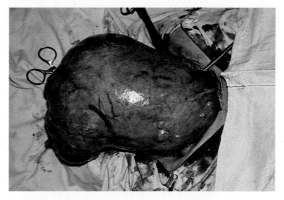

Fig. 115 Enlarged fibroid uterus—operative specimen.

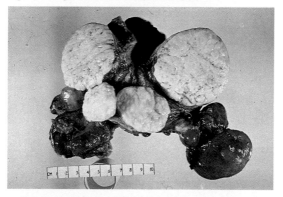

Fig. 116 Calcified fibroids—pathological specimen.

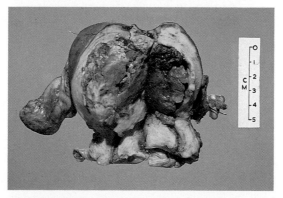

Fig. 117 Pathological specimen of an endometrial carcinoma invading the endometrium.

15 / Benign and malignant conditions of the fallopian tubes

Introduction

The fimbriae of the fallopian tubes pick up the ovum after it is released from the follicle and the cilia of the endosalpinx transport it to the site of fertilization. Sperm are transported by the cilia from the uterine end of the tube laterally to the site of fertilization.

Tubal infection

The tubes can become blocked by infection (or inflammation following trauma). The result of this can be tubal abscess or hydrosalpinx (Fig. 118).

Clinical features

Tubal infection may present with pain of an acute abdomen, especially if an abscess has formed. A hydrosalpinx may be symptomless.

Investigations

Laparoscopy is useful for inspection of the peritoneal aspect of the tubes. Exudate may be seen over the tubes, especially at the fimbriae. If the fimbriae are clubbed, this indicates chronic damage. Fresh and old adhesions may be seen. A hydrosalpinx will be visualized as a swollen tube but not actively infected. In the absence of acute infection, dye can be injected through the cervix. If there is no tubal blockage, filling of the tubes and free spill into the peritoneal cavity can be seen. Hysterosalpingography is a useful investigative technique.

Management

Acute infection should be treated appropriately. Infertility due to tubal damage can be treated by tubal surgery or in vitro fertilization to overcome tubal blockage.

Carcinoma of the fallopian tube

Primary carcinoma of the fallopian tube (Fig. 119) is rare; secondary disease from adjacent structures is more common. The symptoms are classically a watery, bloody vaginal discharge. On examination, an adnexal mass may be felt. The treatment is total abdominal hysterectomy and bilateral oophorectomy.

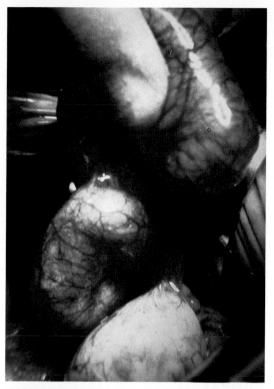

Fig. 118 Hydrosalpinx.

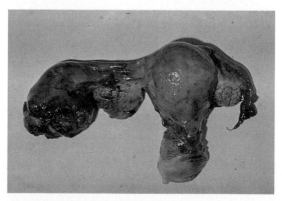

Fig. 119 Carcinoma of the fallopian tube.

16 / Benign and malignant conditions of the ovary

Introduction
Ovarian cysts may be physiological, benign (Fig. 120) or malignant tumours. Ovarian pathology may give rise to symptoms:

- when ovarian enlargement causes pressure on the bladder or rectum
- should the ovary/cyst tort, bleed or rupture causing acute abdominal pain
- should hormonal production be affected.

Physiological cysts (distension cysts)

Clinical types
Follicular cysts: due to enlargement of one or more follicles which fail to rupture. They may be associated with anovulatory cycles, fertility drugs and polycystic ovarian disease. They are usually symptomless and resolve spontaneously.

Corpus luteum cysts: can cause short periods of amenorrhoea followed by heavy vaginal bleeding as the corpus luteum continues to function. Spontaneous resolution is the norm, but intra-abdominal bleeding may cause significant pain.

Endometriomas: result from invagination of endometrial deposits on the surface of the ovary

Polycystic ovaries: enlarged to greater than 2–3 times normal (Fig. 121), with numerous small subcapsular follicular cysts.

Ovarian tumours—benign and malignant

Incidence
Benign tumours of the ovary are common, but the incidence is difficult to determine. Ovarian cancer has an incidence of 14 per 100 000 women in the UK. Each year 5000 new cases are diagnosed and 4000 die from the disease. The incidence of ovarian cancer increases with age, with the peak incidence in the sixties.

Clinical features
Ovarian cancer is often either symptomless or associated with non-specific symptoms such as dyspepsia. A malignant tumour should be suspected in older women, especially if it is fixed, bilateral, rapid-growing or associated with ascites. A solid, or a mixed cystic and solid appearance on ultrasound scanning is also suggestive. In advanced disease there may be venous obstruction of the legs, pain and palpable supraclavicular lymphadenopathy.

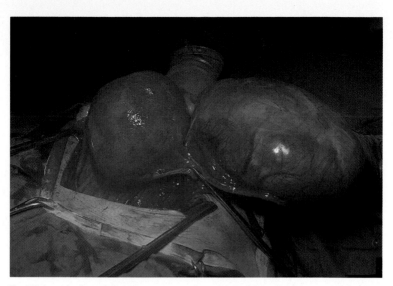

Fig. 120 Large benign ovarian cyst.

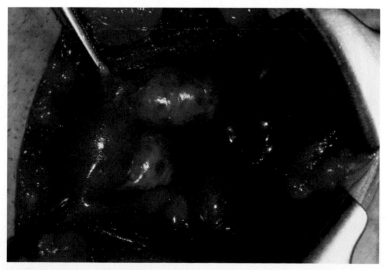

Fig. 121 'Kissing' polycystic ovaries.

Classification   Ovarian tumours can be derived from the following cell types:
- surface epithelium
- germ cells
- gonadal stroma.

Secondary deposits from primary tumours of the breast, stomach, large bowel and uterus may also occur in the ovaries (Krukenberg tumours; Fig. 122).

Tumours derived from surface epithelium
About 90% of ovarian tumours originate from the surface epithelium. These are further subdivided into:
- *serous*, e.g. serous cystadenoma (benign), serous cystadenocarcinoma (malignant, Fig. 123)
- *mucinous*, e.g. mucinous cystadenoma, mucinous cystadenocarcinoma
- *endometrioid*
- *Brenner tumours*
- *clear cell tumours*.

Epithelial ovarian tumours can be benign, of borderline malignancy, or frankly malignant. The malignant forms are collectively known as adenocarcinoma of the ovary.

Tumours derived from germ cells
The germ cells of the ovary are totipotent (i.e. can give rise to various types of tissues). Tumours of germ cells can contain a variety of tissues including teeth, bone, cartilage, muscle, thyroid and nervous tissue. The commonest germ cell tumour is the benign cystic teratoma (dermoid cyst, Fig. 124). These are the commonest tumours in young women. They are bilateral in 10–20% of cases.

Tumours derived from gonadal stroma
Sex cord tumours are rare. Granulosa cell tumours and thecomas secrete oestrogens and can therefore cause precocious puberty in premenarchal girls, and endometrial hyperplasia and post-menopausal bleeding in older women. More than 50% of granulosa cell tumours are malignant; the vast majority of thecomas are benign. Sertoli–Leydig tumours may secrete androgens and can therefore cause progressive virilization.

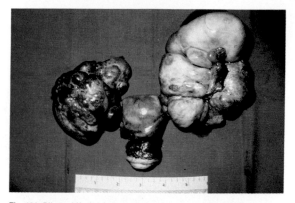

Fig. 122 Bilateral Krukenberg tumours.

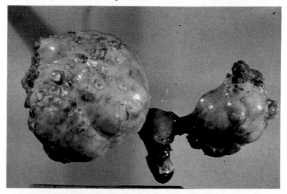

Fig. 123 Serous cystadenocarcinoma.

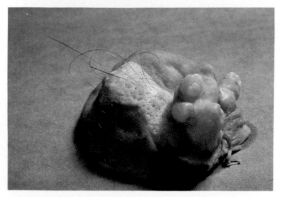

Fig. 124 Benign cystic teratoma.

Management

Benign tumours

If the tumour is greater than 5 cm (Fig. 125), laparotomy should be performed (Fig. 126). Before embarking upon surgery, the risk of malignancy must be assessed to prevent inexperienced operators encountering ovarian cancer with inadequate access through a transverse incision. Enucleation of the cyst may be possible. In older women, total abdominal hysterectomy and bilateral salpingo-oophorectomy are usually performed.

Ovarian cancer

An adequate pre-operative assessment should be made, with a general examination including the breasts and lymph nodes. Laparotomy aims include:

- adequate staging
- removal of tumour and all visible tumour deposits (Figs 127 & 128, p. 100).

Staging requires thorough inspection of the whole abdominal cavity through a vertical incision. Peritoneal washings are taken and the following are either removed or biopsied:

- parietal peritoneum
- omentum
- uterus and other ovary
- bowel and mesentery
- diaphragm
- pelvic and para-aortic lymph nodes.

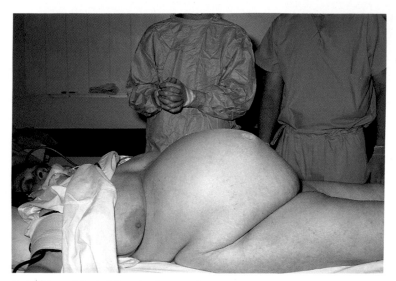
Fig. 125 Gross abdominal distension due to ovarian tumour.

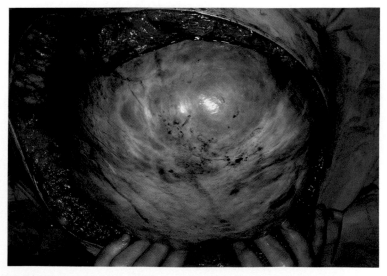
Fig. 126 Laparotomy findings on above.

Staging of ovarian cancer

Stage I: tumour limited to the ovaries.

- Ia Only one ovary involved, no ascites
    - i) capsule not ruptured
    - ii) capsule ruptured.
- Ib Both ovaries involved, no ascites
    - i) capsule not ruptured
    - ii) capsule ruptured.
- Ic One or both ovaries involved with ascites/malignant cells in peritoneal washings.

Stage II: tumour involving one or both ovaries with pelvic extension.

- IIa spread to the uterus and/or tubes
- IIb spread to other pelvic tissues
- IIc as for IIa or IIb with ascites/malignant cells in peritoneal washings.

Stage III: tumour involving one or both ovaries with intra-peritoneal metastases.

State IV: tumour involving one or both ovaries with distant spread.

Surgical measures

In early disease, i.e. stage I, total abdominal hysterectomy, bilateral salpingo-oophorectomy, omentectomy, appendectomy and lymph node biopsy are necessary. Stage Ia(i) and Ib(i) disease require no adjuvant chemotherapy. In younger women with stage Ia disease, who have not completed their family, oophorectomy may be an appropriate short-term measure. In more advanced disease, the aim of surgery is to perform maximum debulking followed by chemotherapy.

Prognosis

The 5-year survival rates for primary ovarian cancer are as follows: Ia 85%, Ib–IIa 40%, IIb 25%, IIc–III 15%, IV < 5%.

The prognosis has changed very little in the last 30 years because women continue to present late in the disease process. Effective screening would be of value if it were possible to detect disease in its early stages, thereby enabling more effective treatment. Ultrasound scanning and various tumour markers (e.g. CA 125) are being evaluated for future use.

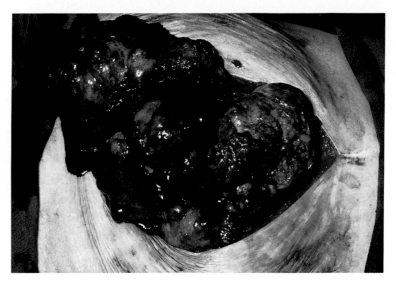

Fig. 127 Disseminated ovarian adenocarcinoma.

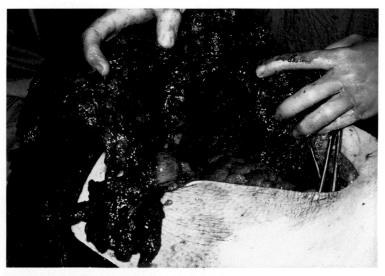

Fig. 128 Omental infiltration with ovarian adenocarcinoma.

17 / **The menopause and climacteric**

Definition   The menopause is a woman's last menstrual period; the climacteric is the period of ovarian decline which includes the menopause.

Aetiology   At the beginning of the climacteric, the remaining ovarian follicles become increasingly resistant to gonadotrophin stimulation, and so more gonadotrophins are produced in response to the decreasing oestrogen levels.

Pathology   Atrophy occurs in all tissues that are sensitive to oestrogen, especially the urogenital system, breasts, and skin.

Changes can also occur in bony tissue. Osteoporosis is defined as a decreased amount of bony tissue per unit volume of bone, leading to structural weakness. With lowered oestrogen levels there appears to be a decrease in osteoblast function and an increase in bone resorption. This leads to a structural weakness in bone and increases the risk of fracture. The commonest sites of fracture are the radius, the neck of the femur and the vertebral spine (Fig. 129).

Cardiovascular disease also increases with the lowered oestrogen levels of the menopause. An increase in total cholesterol and low-density lipoprotein cholesterol occurs, along with a decline in high-density lipoprotein. While these lipid changes account for increased risk, other factors such as changes in glucose tolerance and the direct effects of oestrogen on arterial and venous blood flow are likely to be important.

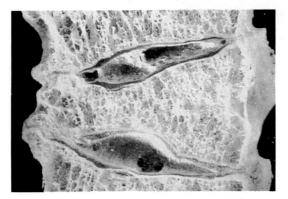

Fig. 129 Post mortem specimen of osteoporotic wedge fracture.

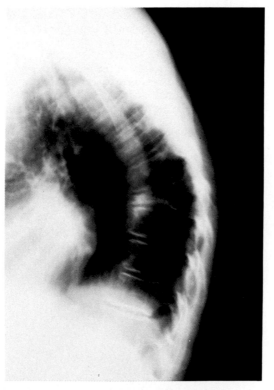

Fig. 130 X-ray showing wedge fracture of thoracic spine.

Clinical features   Hot flushes and night sweats are the classical symptoms of the menopause. Other symptoms include depression, vaginal soreness, vaginal dryness, urinary frequency, headaches and joint pains. On examination, hair loss, dry skin and vaginal atrophy may be present.

Osteoporosis is described as the 'silent epidemic' in that the disease may not be detected until the woman falls and fractures her osteoporotic bone(s). Wedge fractures of the spine may be detected on X-ray (Fig. 130, p. 102) and, if multiple, may produce the 'dowager's hump'.

Investigations   If the diagnosis is in doubt, an FSH level of greater than 15 i.u./l will confirm ovarian failure.

Noninvasive methods are now available to assess bone density. Single photon absorptiometry was initially used, then dual photon, and now dual energy X-rays are used as the radioactive source (DEXA, Fig. 131). Bone densitometry results of the hip are shown in Figure 132.

Blood pressure, breasts and cervical cytology should be checked as indicated. Mammography may be offered routinely in the future to menopausal women.

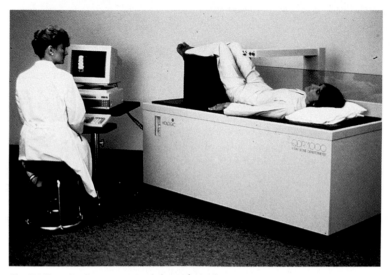

Fig. 131 Bone density measurement being performed.

Nuclear Medicine Dept. Guy's Hospital

k = 1.245   d0 = 102.6(1.000)[1]

92 x 113

Hologic QDR 1000 (S/N 122)
Version 3.20
Left Hip

A1012880E	Wed Oct 12 16:08 1988		
Name:			
Comment:			
I.D.:		Sex:	F
S.S.#:	– –	Ethnic:	C
ZIP Code:		Height:5' 9"	
Scan Code:		Weight:	77
BirthDate:	01/01/61	Age:	27
Physician:	FOGELMAN		

C.F.	0.996	1.031	1.000
	FOR INVESTIGATIONAL USE ONLY		
Region	Area (cm2)	BMC (grams)	BMD (gms/cm2)
Neck	4.62	4.63	1.003
Troch	10.79	9.28	0.860
Inter	16.22	19.92	1.228
TOTAL	31.63	33.83	1.070
Ward's	0.96	0.81	0.840
Midline (100,118)–(164, 58)			
Neck	−53 x	14 at [27, 9]	
Troch	−2 x	44 at [0, 0]	
Ward's	−11 x	11 at [13, 11]	

HOLOGIC

Fig. 132 DEXA printout of bone density.

Management   Hormone replacement therapy is the most appropriate treatment for women with menopause-related problems.

The indications are:

- menopause related symptoms, early menopause,
- osteoporosis and cardiovascular protection.

Contraindications are breast carcinoma, endometrial carcinoma and liver disease.

There are various methods of administration (Fig. 133).

Oral. Oestrogen tablets are given continuously and progestogen tablets are given for 12 days of each calendar month. Various tablets are being developed to provide continuous oestrogen and progesterone, thus alleviating the monthly bleeding. Women who do not have a uterus do not need progestogen.

Parenteral. Patches can be placed on the skin to deliver a constant dose of oestrogen. Oestrogen creams can be used on the skin or intravaginally. Oestradiol implants (Fig. 134) can be inserted subcutaneously every 6 months; a testosterone implant may be inserted at the same time if the woman is sexually active, to improve libido.

With all the above preparations, progestogens must be given if there is a uterus.

Complications   HRT has been connected with an increased risk of carcinoma. These claims are largely unfounded, although there may be a small increased risk of carcinoma of the breast with prolonged therapy, i.e. after 10 years.

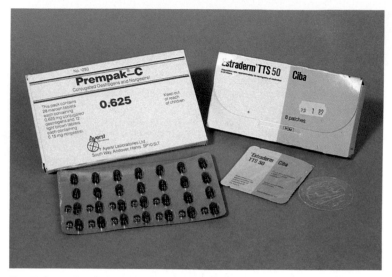

Fig. 133 Preparations for hormone replacement therapy.

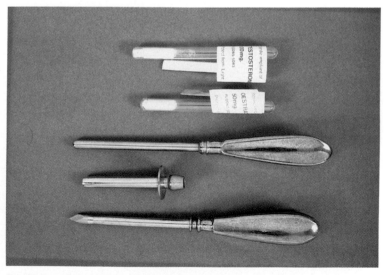

Fig. 134 Testosterone and oestradiol implants.

18 / **Uterovaginal prolapse**

Anatomical considerations The anterior vaginal wall is supported by the pubocervical fascia. This extends from the back of the symphysis pubis to the cervix and upper vagina. The posterior vaginal wall is supported by fibrous tissue of the rectovaginal septum and the levator ani muscles. The uterus is supported mainly by the cardinal or transverse cervical ligaments which merge with the uterosacral ligaments before joining the cervix.

Definition Uterovaginal prolapse is the downward displacement of the uterus and/or vagina towards or through the introitus. The bladder, urethra, rectum and bowel may also be involved.

Three degrees of uterine prolapse are described:

- *1st degree*—descent of the cervix to the introitus.
- *2nd degree*—descent of the cervix but not the whole uterus through the introitus.
- *3rd degree*—(procidentia; Fig. 135)—descent of the cervix and whole uterus through the introitus.

Vaginal wall prolapse

A prolapse of the lowest one-third of the anterior vagina involves the urethra and is called a urethrocoele. Prolapse of the upper two-thirds of the anterior vaginal wall involves the bladder and is therefore called a cystocoele (Fig. 136). When the lower portion of the posterior vaginal wall prolapses, it brings with it the rectum and is therefore termed a rectocoele. Prolapse of the vaginal wall above this involves the Pouch of Douglas. This type of herniation is called an enterocoele.

Aetiology Prolapse is uncommon in nulliparous women. In these cases it is due to congenital weakness of the pelvic-supporting structures. The majority of women with prolapse have had children. Childbirth is associated with damage to the ligamentous tissues of the pelvis and nerve supply of the pelvic floor muscles causing later weakness. Other factors contributing to or exacerbating these effects include postmenopausal atrophy of pelvic-supporting tissue and chronic raised intra-abdominal pressure e.g. with obesity or chronic cough.

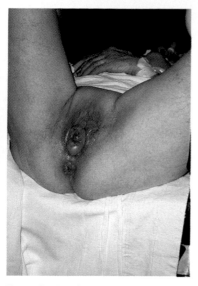

Fig. 135 Procidentia.

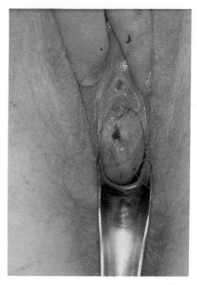

Fig. 136 Cystocoele.

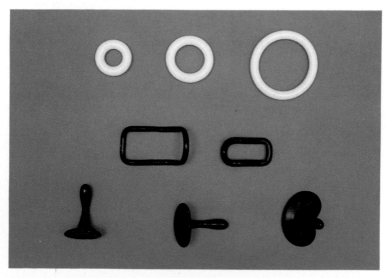

Fig. 137 Rings and shelf pessaries used to relieve prolapse.

Clinical features   Patients may describe a feeling of something 'coming down', and there is the presence of a lump protruding through the vulva. Urinary incontinence may be associated with a urethrocoele. Urinary retention may be seen when a large cystocoele is present. Difficulty with defaecation may also be present. Pain is not a feature of prolapse, but dragging discomfort and backache which worsen throughout the day may be experienced.

Management   **Prophylaxis.** Avoid traumatic vaginal deliveries and encourage antenatal and postnatal pelvic floor exercises. Discourage cigarette smoking and use hormone replacement therapy appropriately in post-menopausal women.

Conservative treatment. Rings and shelf pessaries (Fig. 137, p. 108) are a suitable short-term option in women unfit or not keen to undergo surgery, and between pregnancies.

Surgery. Procedures include the following.

- *Anterior repair* corrects a cystocoele, but may not be the most appropriate treatment for stress incontinence.
- *Posterior repair* corrects a rectocoele.
- *Vaginal hysterectomy* is the treatment of choice in uterine prolapse and is combined with anterior and posterior repairs as necessary (Fig. 138).
- *Manchester (Fothergill) repair* involves shortening the transverse cervical ligaments and amputating the cervix, together with an anterior repair. It is a useful operation when the uterine body is well supported, but the cervix is elongated and protruding.

Complications   Long-term use of pessaries can cause vaginal ulceration. Immediate complications of vaginal surgery include haemorrhage, haematoma formation, infection and urinary retention. Wound breakdown and extrusion of bowel through the vagina (Fig. 139) are extremely rare. In the longer term, stenosis and dyspareunia may result. Prolapse may also recur.

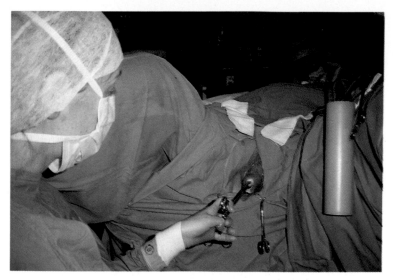

Fig. 138 Procidentia at commencement of vaginal hysterectomy.

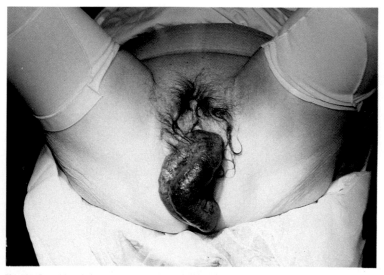

Fig. 139 Bowel herniation—a rare complication of vaginal hysterectomy.

19 / Urinary incontinence

Genuine stress incontinence

Definition Involuntary loss of urine when intra-abdominal pressure rises.

Aetiology Urethral sphincter weakness which is either congenital or secondary to multiparity, prolapse, menopause or previous surgery.

Clinical features The patient gives a history of losing urine involuntarily when she laughs, coughs or sneezes. On examination the vulva may be excoriated due to persistent wetness. If the patient is placed in the Sim's position and a Sim's speculum is inserted to display the anterior vaginal wall, urine loss may be demonstrated when the patient is asked to cough (providing her bladder is not empty). A cystocoele may be present.

Investigations A mid-stream urine specimen should be taken for microscopy and culture. If there is any suggestion of a 'mixed' picture, i.e. symptoms of urge as well as stress, urodynamic investigations are essential. Padweighing can be used to assess incontinence (Fig. 140). Videocysto-urethography (Fig. 141, & Fig. 142, p.114) is also useful.

Management Infection should be treated. Other treatments include:
- *Colposuspension*. The bladder neck is elevated by inserting sutures beside the urethra and bladder neck.
- *Anterior colporraphy*. The urethra is elevated from below after opening up the anterior vaginal wall.
- *Slings*. Organic or inorganic material is used.
- *Endoscopic bladder neck suspensions*. This is useful for recurrent stress incontinence.
- *Artificial sphincters*.
- *Physiotherapy* involving pelvic floor exercises with or without Faradism is also used for mild cases, or where surgery is contraindicated.

Complications Following surgery, voiding difficulties are common and recurrence of the stress incontinence is not uncommon. The results of surgery are poor if detrusor instability was present originally.

Prognosis Colposuspensions have a 90% cure rate, and anterior colporraphies 40–60%.

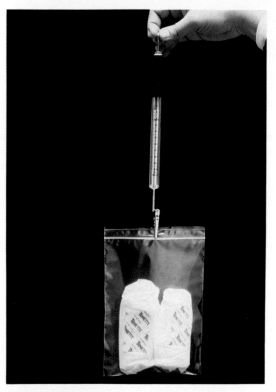

Fig. 140 Pad weighing to assess incontinence.

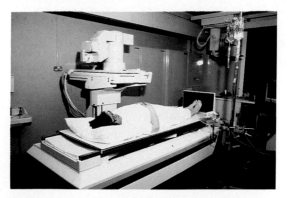

Fig. 141 Videocystourethography in progress.

Urge incontinence

Definition

Involuntary loss of urine caused by uninhibited detrusor contractions.

Aetiology

Most cases are idiopathic. The detrusor contracts in an uninhibited fashion causing urgency and frequency, and when the intravesical pressure exceeds the intraurethral pressure, incontinence results.

Clinical features

The history will reveal urinary frequency, urgency, nocturia and, perhaps, incontinence. On examination there is usually no abnormality.

Investigations

Midstream urine (MSU). Infection can produce the same symptoms.

Urodynamics. Subtracted cystometry will show uninhibited detrusor contractions during bladder filling (Fig. 143).

Management

Bladder drill. This requires patient motivation and ideally biofeedback. The patient is told to pass urine at certain time intervals which are then gradually increased until 3 or 4 hours is reached.

Drug therapy. Calcium antagonists, anticholinergic agents, ganglion blockers, oestrogen replacement, and postganglion blockers.

Surgery. Clam cystoplasty, bladder transection and sacral neurectomy are rarely used and are reserved for difficult cases.

Complications

Recurrence of symptoms is common. Bladder rupture can occur with cystodistension. Voiding difficulties can occur after surgery.

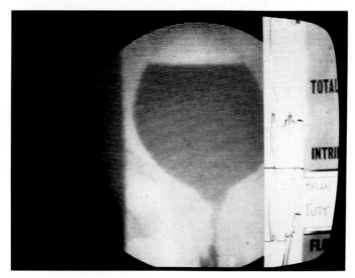

Fig. 142 Leakage of urine into bladder neck seen on videocystourethography.

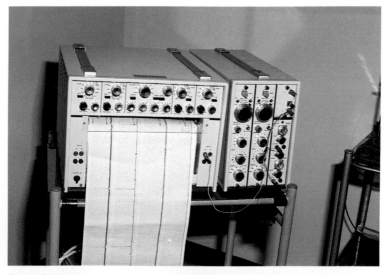

Fig. 143 Cystometry readout showing a stable bladder.

Overflow incontinence

Definition Frequent involuntary loss of small volumes of urine, slow urinary stream, and a post-micturition feeling of incomplete emptying.

Aetiology Obstruction to bladder outflow in bladder atony which can be due to motor neuron lesions, drugs, surgery, pelvic mass, uterovaginal prolapse, local inflammation or immobilization.

Clinical features History will reveal the above symptoms. Examination will demonstrate an enlarged bladder, and catheterization will produce a large residual volume of urine.

Investigations **MSU**

Cystometry. This will demonstrate a delayed first sensation and a large bladder capacity. Maximum voiding pressure will be normal or increased, and the peak flow rate will be slow.

Micturating cystourethrogram (Fig. 144).

Uroflowmeter (Fig. 145).

Treatment This will depend on the cause. Neurological causes are not treatable and intermittent self-catheterisation can be learnt.

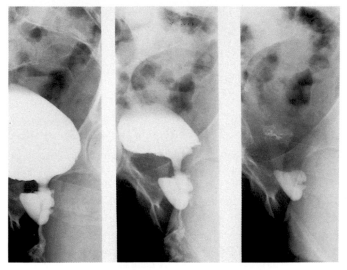

Fig. 144 Micturating cystogram demonstrating large urethral diverticulum.

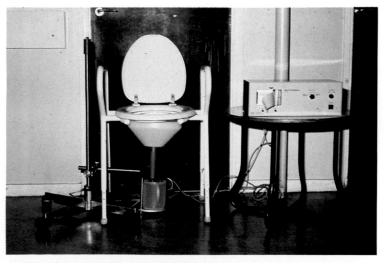

Fig. 145 Uroflowmeter used to assess urinary flow.

True incontinence

Definition Continuous incontinence.

Aetiology Usually due to a fistulous track (Fig. 146) secondary to obstructed labour, surgery, carcinoma, or radiotherapy.

Clinical features There will be a history of continuous draining of urine from vagina. Examination may reveal the track, and colouring the urine may aid location (Fig. 147).

Investigations A micturating cystourethrogram and/or an IVP may help location.

Management **Conservative:** depending on aetiology, some may heal with time.

Surgery: can be performed abdominally or vaginally. The fistulous track is removed and an interposition graft may be used if the tissues are poor.

Complications Stress incontinence, vaginal scarring and recurrence.

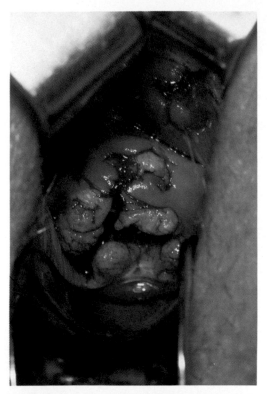

Fig. 146 Bladder mucosa visible through irregular fragments of vaginal mucosa.

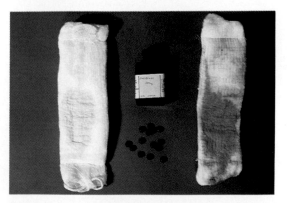

Fig. 147 Pyridium tablets can be used to colour urine.

Index

cx